Library of Congress Cataloging in Publication Data

Puetz, Belinda E.
Continuing education for nurses.

Includes bibliographies and index.
1. Nursing—Study and teaching (Continuing education).
I. Peters, Faye L.
II. Title.

RT76.P83          610.73'0715          81-2830
ISBN: 0-89443-373-3                    AACR2

Copyright © 1981 Aspen Systems Corporation

All rights reserved. This book, or parts thereof, may not be
reproduced in any form or by any means, electronic or
mechanical, including photocopy, recording, or any
information storage and retrieval system now known or
to be invented, without written permission from the
publisher, except in the case of brief quotations embodied
in critical articles or reviews. For information, address
Aspen Systems Corporation, 1600 Research Boulevard,
Rockville, Maryland 20850.

Library of Congress Catalog Card Number: 81-2830
ISBN: 0-89443-373-3

*Printed in the United States of America*

1  2  3  4  5

# CONTINUING EDUCATIO FOR NURSES

## A Complete Guide to Effective Progra

**Belinda E. Puetz, R.N., Ph.D.**
Director of Continuing Education
Indiana State Nurses' Association
Indianapolis, Indiana

**Faye L. Peters, R.N., M. S.Ed.**
Coordinator of Continuing Education in Nursing
Indiana University—Purdue University at Indianapolis,
Columbus Campus
Columbus, Indiana

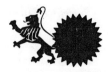

AN ASPEN PUBLICATION®
Aspen Systems Corporation
Rockville, Maryland
London
1981

LANSING COMMUNITY COLLEGE LIBRARY

*To Our Parents*

# Table of Contents

# Foreword

During the 1970s, continuing education in nursing has expanded explosively, fueled by government legislation, professional organization standards and requirements, regulatory bodies such as the Joint Commission on Accreditation of Hospitals, societal pressures for improved health care delivery, and the demands of nurses seeking to provide health care responsive to societal needs.

These demands give rise to the need for educators to provide quality continuing education and staff development activities designed to assist nurses to function as competent practitioners in a variety of settings. The demand for proficient continuing and staff development educators greatly exceeds the supply. As a result, nurses lacking knowledge of how to organize and implement quality educational offerings effectively for adult learners have been placed in these positions. All too frequently, these nurses have experienced the frustrations associated with the Peter Principle—the facetious proposition that employees tend to be promoted until they reach their level of incompetence.

Furthermore, the field of continuing education for professionals has evolved slowly but consistently into a discipline possessing a differentiated body of knowledge related to organizational structure, principles of planning for education activities, teaching strategies, selection and utilization of materials and resources, evaluation, and research. In essence, continuing and staff development educators are assuming the role of stage managers by setting the stage and shifting the scenery to provide an enriched educational environment for adult learners in nursing. This emerging role requires new competencies for continuing education practitioners.

By virtue of their own distinguished roles in continuing education in nursing, the authors use an experiential approach in developing this primer for those new to the field of continuing education and staff development. The work provides excellent "how-to" information to assist beginners to function effectively in their newly emerging roles as continuing and staff development educators. In addition, the book's comprehensive scope serves as a valuable reference resource for seasoned educators seeking assistance in expanding their proficiencies in specific areas.

In keeping with the primer orientation of this book, readers will find it helpful as they confront the issues, problems, concerns, and frustrations of daily practice to refer to the appropriate chapters for assistance on the specific concerns. Readers will find that this book is an indispensable, quick reference tool to have handy as problems arise from time to time.

Whatever the problem, *Continuing Education for Nurses: A Complete Guide to Effective Programs* will provide authentic, practical information; intellectual challenges; and professional stimulation for educators and leaders. The authors have opened the door—the challenge now is that of the readers.

JEAN E. SCHWEER

*Professor of Nursing*
*Assistant Dean, Continuing Education in Nursing*
*Indiana University School of Nursing*
*Indianapolis, Indiana*

# Preface

*Learning follows various roads,*
*We note the start but not the end.*
*For Time and Fate must rule the course,*
*While we see not beyond the bend.*
*Kahlil Gibran*

This book is intended to provide a beginning for learning about continuing education and staff development. The idea and motivation to undertake developing a primer in this field came from our attendance at many national conferences on continuing education in nursing. From the very first such annual gathering, the continuing educators and persons in staff development who were present identified their need for "how-to" information. Beginning practitioners in this field have few resources for practical application of knowledge and skills.

In our years as continuing educators we also have struggled with some of those needs. We also were beginners and sought help from our more experienced colleagues. As we grew more proficient in planning, implementing, evaluating, and approving continuing education activities, we were able to attain a comfort and competence level that we now seek to share with others.

It is our hope that by providing you, the reader, with the benefit of our experience, you will find the road a bit easier to travel.

BELINDA E. PUETZ, R.N., PH.D.
FAYE L. PETERS, R.N., M.S.ED.
July 1981

# Chapter 1

# Overview of the Principles of Adult Education

Those in continuing education and staff development are responsible for programming and teaching for adults and must know and use the concepts of adult education. For the authors' purposes, adults are defined as persons who have completed the basic program that has prepared them to practice their profession. Their continuing education is for the purpose of updating their knowledge and skills or preparing them to practice in a different setting or a different area of expertise. Underlying professional continuing education is the need to improve the health care of the public.

## LIFELONG LEARNING

Lifelong learning is not a new concept either in general or in nursing. A great deal of incidental learning always has been a part of the day-to-day work of practicing nurses. Some nurses have continued their education throughout their careers for their own self-satisfaction and from the desire to be better practitioners. Many have continued their education on a formal basis to achieve the baccalaureate degree in nursing if their basic preparation was completed in a diploma or associate degree program. Increasing numbers are continuing their education beyond the basic programs to complete graduate programs. The concept of continuing education in nursing through nonacademic offerings expanded substantially in the late 60s and throughout the 70s. According to the American Nurses' Association, these offerings "consist of planned, organized learning experiences designed to augment the knowledge, skills and attitudes of registered nurses for the enhancement of nursing practice, education, administration, and research to the end of improving health care to the public."[1]

The first national conference for continuing educators in nursing was held in 1969 and resulted eventually in the establishment of the Council on Con-

1

tinuing Education within the American Nurses' Association. Through this council, standards for continuing education were established and an accreditation process implemented. The council also has provided opportunities for educators to share common problems and look for solutions to such problems as the evaluation of programs in nursing and the use of nontraditional learning techniques. The activities of the council and the resulting standards are built on the concept of lifelong learning and of the principles of adult education in planning, implementing, and evaluating continuing courses in nursing.

The importance of lifelong learning is being given increasing emphasis in basic nursing programs. Statements of beliefs about nurses' responsibilities in continuing their education, maintaining their competence, and having up-to-date knowledge and skills are being included in philosophies of basic nursing programs. These statements in philosophies on concepts of learning that are influenced by past experiences, acquired knowledge, current perception of need, and independence reflect the beliefs of adult education.

## WHY LIFELONG LEARNING IN NURSING?

The need for lifelong learning in nursing is rather easy to substantiate, as it is for most professional groups. The changes that have occurred, and continue to take place, in the delivery of health care and the changing role of nurses in that system are sufficient evidence that learning is a continuing process. Nursing is influenced by socioeconomic changes, policy developments in the political arena, and the vast technological advances in the health care field.

Some of the socioeconomic changes have had an impact on the number of persons now eligible to receive health care and the methods by which payment will be made for them. These changes have imposed increasing demands in terms of not only the numbers of nurses required but also the types of skills they will need in a variety of settings for health care delivery. The emphasis on prevention to avoid the costly treatments in an acute care facility requires nurses to have a good knowledge base in illness prevention and to be skilled in teaching consumers about health care. The changing age of the population requires nurses skilled in gerontology.

Policies developed at both governmental and nongovernmental levels have a definite impact on the knowledge and skills required of nurses. The increased concern about cost containment and reimbursement policies for payment of health care require nurses, particularly in management positions, to know more about budgeting and staffing to get the maximum utilization of personnel at the least expense. Policies on determining the necessity for admission of a patient for a particular level of care, and length of stay, require that nurses do better planning for the care both in the facility and after discharge.

The standards that facilities must meet for accrediting bodies can have an impact on the way nursing is practiced and can require new knowledge and skills.

Technology has been a major force in the need for lifelong learning for nurses and in the design of courses to prepare them for specialty areas. Not only is more technology being used in nursing, but it is becoming increasingly complex. This requires in-depth courses to prepare nurses to work in specialized units such as critical care for adults and children, transplants, and surgery. The use of computers in health care delivery is requiring nurses to acquire basic knowledge and skill in this technology. The vast array of new treatment methods and drugs involved mean that nurses must be constant learners.

Continuing education must respond to the needs of nurses practicing under these increased demands. More continuing education programs are being made available to help nurses learn to deal with the many stresses of their work environment and to cope with the more personal needs that together are a crucial part of lifelong learning.

## PURPOSES OF LIFELONG LEARNING IN NURSING

Nurses attend continuing education activities for a variety of purposes. It is important for continuing educators to consider their program's mission in determining what purposes it can achieve and what other resources it may need to help nurses in achieving their learning needs.

In analyzing the "why" of professional development, Preston P. LeBreton, Professor of Management and Organization at the University of Washington, discusses awareness strategies that can be useful in determining the purpose of continuing education for a professional group. He describes those strategies in three broad time frames: (1) anticipatory, (2) concurrent, (3) after the fact.[2] He declares:

"An anticipatory strategy suggests that the planners study the future developmental needs of their clients as much as possible before the fact. Learning experiences then can be made available to professionals to allow them to maintain their competence throughout their productive lifetimes without experiencing periods of reduced effectiveness and efficiency."[3] Continuing education has found this difficult to accomplish in terms of the number of nurses and the many other circumstances that can impede long-range planning, such as the effort to bring all nurses up-to-date with changes, change in policies, and procedures that were not expected and could not be planned ahead of time. Through curriculum planning, efforts are being directed toward studying the predictions about health care, social trends, population trends, and the many other factors that influence how nurses practice. However, this requires the continuing education staff to have the time to use an anticipatory approach and calls for a nurse population interested in acquiring knowledge and skills for future use. Continuing education departments, particularly in colleges and universities, need support for research, for staff to monitor research findings in health care and nursing, and to seek new methods for disseminating these findings so the anticipatory approach to lifelong learning can accomplish its objectives.

"A concurrent strategy is tied to significant changes in job demand. A training or education need would be identified whenever a professional is asked to take on a new or expanded assignment which requires additional qualifications."[4]

Concurrent strategies can be used, particularly by staff development departments, in preparing nurses for changes being planned for the health care facility. For example, if the institution plans to start intensive care units for high-risk infants, the staff development department can anticipate the type of educational experiences that nurses on this unit will need and determine how to provide appropriate courses. If the college or university program is aware of anticipated needs in a health care facility, it can plan ways to assist the institution in meeting those requirements before the change is made. The program also can cope with new job demands in timely fashion. One purpose of continuing education is to prepare nurses for career changes. This may involve their moving from a generalized medical-surgical unit to a special care unit or from staff nurse to a managerial role requiring different skills.

LeBreton's "after-the-fact awareness strategy" is "characterized by an identification of education or training needs after an individual or group has demonstrated repeatedly a significant inability to cope with work requirements or opportunities."[5] When situations occur that nurses feel unable to handle or when seemingly unsolvable problems exist, nurses are more likely to attend a course or workshop that they identify as providing the potential for helping to solve the problem or gain the knowledge or skill in which they perceive they are deficient. Groups of nurses may request continuing education or staff development programs to plan offerings when they perceive a need.

Continuing education opportunities should be provided under all three strategies to meet the differing needs of the nurse population. Nurses, like other professionals, must have opportunities to keep up with changes in the field (which provides an important role for their professional associations). Continuing education also enhances the opportunity for nurses to maintain a fresh outlook on their practice and to retain the ability to learn. As Cyril Houle, Professor emeritus at the University of Chicago, states, "the skills of mastering knowledge are like other skills—they are learned with practice, they atrophy from disuse and they can later be regained only with difficulty."[6] This may be the most important purpose of lifelong learning.

## ADULT LEARNERS

Philosophies for continuing education activities in nursing usually contain statements that reflect the belief that these programs are built on principles of adult education. Such statements as "the planned learning experiences are built upon adult education principles" and "we believe that adults are self-directed, problem oriented and possess varied competencies as a result of life experiences" reflect the importance of recognizing the principles of adult education in nursing.

With these philosophical beliefs as a basis, all persons involved in planning, conducting, and evaluating these events must be familiar with and use concepts of adult education. Adult learners have specific characteristics that must be known and understood by teachers and continuing education staffs. These persons should be able to relate these concepts to the nurses who participate.

The readiness to learn is a long-held concept that applies to children as well as adults. "It is well known that educational development occurs best through sequencing of learning activities into developmental tasks so that the learner is presented with opportunities for learning certain topics or activities when he is 'ready' to assimilate them, not before."[7] For example, basic nursing students are required to take physical, biological, and social sciences early in the curriculum so that the principles of these courses can be used in the professional nursing courses. Students must complete prescribed courses and experiences to meet requirements for graduation.

Nurses attending continuing education offerings no longer are concerned about meeting requirements for graduation. They are concerned about how learning experiences and their own perceived needs relate to the practice of their profession. Their readiness to learn and willingness to participate in a learning situation is related directly to what they perceive as an interest or need. Professionals who encounter work situations that they feel unable to handle are much more likely to be ready to learn than those attending at the direction of someone else. As mandatory continuing education requirements for relicensure are enacted in more states, some nurses may be attending the courses to meet those requirements rather than to meet an identified need or interest. The continuing education counselor becomes more important in assisting these nurses in making choices for the courses they will take. Persons who are "sent" to educational offerings without having expressed either a need or an interest present a challenge to teachers and staff. These individuals do not enter the course ready to learn and may leave without having learned anything. (Dealing with this problem is discussed in the section on teaching adults later in this chapter.)

## The Self-Concept Factor

Adults enter the learning setting with a strong self-concept. They have spent years deciding who they are and what they can do. They feel capable of self-direction, including making decisions about what and how they need to learn. They have built this self-concept through their childhood and adult years on the basis of previous learning, accomplishments, and experiences in living and working. Nurses bring to the classes self-concepts that are related directly to their experiences in their profession as well as the status of the positions they have achieved on the job. They are accustomed to making decisions about their own lives as well as about the health care given to others. They are faced constantly with making decisions, frequently very critical ones.

Adults view themselves as mature, independent persons. They expect to be treated as individuals who still maintain the power to control what happens to them. They expect that they will be treated with respect and that their dignity and self-esteem will be protected. Adults are not likely to remain in an activity that is a threat to their self-esteem or in which they are treated as children.

It is important to note that nurses in continuing education have not always had experience in assuming responsibility for directing their own learning. Their past educational experiences may not have allowed for self-direction and initially they may be uncomfortable when they find themselves in situations where they are expected to be involved in (1) defining the objectives for the learning experience, (2) being active participants, and/or (3) making decisions related to the course content. Learners vary in the degree of responsibility they are willing to assume for their education. Teachers in continuing education must be aware of learners' expectations that the educators are totally responsible for the class experience and must help the nurses in becoming active participants.

Closely related to adults' self-concept are the experiences they have had. Unlike children in a learning situation, adults have had opportunities to gain more experience based on the number of years they have lived and the responsibilities they have had to assume. They have had opportunities for a wider variety of experiences through education, work, and social contacts. Nurses come with different types of work experience. Through this career work they also have gained much experience in dealing with different types of people and situations. The world of adults is much wider than that of children, requiring adults to function in different roles in the family, in the community, and in the world of work. The amount and variety of adults' experiences are important resources to be shared with others in class. The participants learn from each other, based on their sharing of experiences.

Past experiences also form a rich foundation on which to base new ones and to relate new learning to past activities. The learners' most valuable resources are their own experiences.

Perhaps no other characteristic of adults is more evident than that of their time perspective. Nurses are interested in continuing education that can be applied immediately to their work situation. They want learning activities that are of use in their role as doers in the work world. The "here and now" application of learning is a key ingredient for continuing education in nursing.

## Learning Styles

Adults have a problem-solving orientation in learning rather than just being concerned about the content of the courses. They want to have the opportunity to seek solutions to situations in their work. The way they approach these solutions is highly individualized and may or may not be the most effective method. They may require assistance in learning to be more effective in problem solving, particularly in taking the time necessary to identify and define the issue and seek alternative ways for dealing with it. They may be seeking solutions from others without taking the time to go through the process of solving the problem for themselves.

Adults have developed different learning styles and respond accordingly in the class situation. Some persons learn best in action-oriented, participative courses. Others may be more dependent on the information provided by the teacher, who must use a variety of methods to accommodate these differences.

Adult learners are fearful of making mistakes or being exposed to failure in the presence of others. They need to be allowed to make a choice about participating in an activity, such as role playing, if they are uncomfortable about their ability to perform. The learner who expresses concern about "making a fool of myself" obviously is uncomfortable with the situation and not ready to risk participating. Different arrangements may be necessary for this individual, or the passage of time may enable the person to develop a level of comfort that will permit participation. By minimizing the learner's mistakes and praising achievement, the fear of making a mistake or looking stupid can be lessened. It also is important to assist adults to evaluate their strengths honestly, which also can assist them in building self-confidence and reduce the fear of failure.

Adult learners have developed value systems that are shaped by family background, personal experiences, and the environmental setting in which they live. These factors also shape their personality. Their values and their personalities cannot be divorced from their learning experience. Students (nurses) should not be made to feel uncomfortable in class because of their values, interests, or personalities.

Adults are more secure in situations that provide some structure and in which they can visualize the goals. They also are more comfortable when they can see a logical pattern and structure that will enable the goals to be achieved. Learning experiences should proceed in a logical sequence and at a comfortable pace. Students need to have information summarized at intervals and determine how they are progressing toward the goal.

Change cannot be forced on people, who need time to assimilate information and discover its meaning. Only after they have been able to acquire meaning on their own terms can they apply and use the information. Learning situations not only need to provide time for individuals to examine issues and ideas but also need to give them a sense of the teacher's helping relationship. Individuals need a feeling of acceptance from both the teacher and classmates and to feel free to express ideas without fear of criticism. A sense of acceptance and respect as a group member will encourage others in the class to share. Learners must understand that there is a difference between acceptance and agreement. Acceptance indicates a willingness to listen without having to concur with the ideas or beliefs being expressed. Agreement means going along with others' ideas. This is not necessarily productive in a learning group. Disagreement can provide challenges to the group. Learners are seeking acceptance and the right to change as they themselves perceive a need to change.

Adult learners are potential change agents. In understanding the use of problem-solving approaches, they are learning how to distinguish between causes and symptoms. This knowledge is essential for the change agent. Learners need to be assisted in acquiring change techniques that will enable them to return to their jobs not only with new knowledge and skill but also with abilities that will help in taking actions that will incorporate the use of this knowledge. A continuing education course should include opportunities for nurses to learn how to introduce change in the work setting.

The proper atmosphere in the educational setting will enable individuals to gain a greater trust in themselves to contribute to their own learning, to assist others in this process, and to make changes in their practice. They begin to realize the inner resources they have to draw on in determining the meaning and relevance of continuing education. They become more independent in their thinking and rely less on the teachers for all the information. They are able to draw on past experiences to give meaning to new ones. Educational experience should build learners' self-confidence and self-esteem.

## THE LEARNING ENVIRONMENT

All persons who work with adults in education must be cognizant of the characteristics of the individuals in order to know best how to approach the activity. The teacher plays a key role in creating the climate that will enable the adult to have a meaningful learning experience.

The learning environment, physiological and psychological, is crucial if learning is to take place. Both the teacher and the administrator should be aware of the environmental factors that can facilitate learning.

## Psychological Environment

The psychological environment is established for the activity by the staff or teacher in initiating efforts to make the learner feel comfortable on arrival for the educational activity. The learner is greeted and provided with essential information such as a name tag, handout materials, and seating information. If possible, learners should be introduced to their fellow learners as they arrive. Nurses frequently are uncomfortable entering a classroom with a group they do not know and need the support of others. Learners should feel accepted as individuals, a feeling that can be achieved best when they sense they are being accepted at the beginning of the session.

The ground rules must be established as a part of the introduction. The teacher recognizes that learning is a process that is controlled by the student, not the instructor. This should be shared with the learners to help them understand the educator's role as a facilitator in assisting them in processing information provided by the teacher and their classmates and discover the meaning of this material for themselves. The relevancy of the content to their own work situation or personal life is a determination they must make with assistance from the teacher and classmates.

Learners need to be oriented to the concept that education is a shared process requiring cooperation and collaboration with their classmates and the teachers. Teachers of adults also enter the course expecting to learn from the students. It is important that this feeling is shared early in setting the ground rules so teacher and learner will have the same understanding of expectations of each other. This encourages learners to become active participants, gives recognition to the contributions that they have to share with each other and the teacher, and creates an atmosphere that stimulates exchanges of ideas.

## Freedom of Ideas

The teacher establishes an atmosphere in which learners know that there is room for differences in ideas that not only are acceptable but also are desirable in the exploration of the subject and in solving problems. Nurses should be encouraged to feel free in expressing their own opinions and in exploring these with others in the group. The group should understand that openness is essential in the learning process and that individuals need to feel they can express an idea or opinion without the fear of being made to feel stupid, humiliated, or embarrassed by the others. This is an essential part of the psychological atmosphere needed for the learning situation.

An open atmosphere also requires a feeling of trust and respect. The teacher of adults in continuing education establishes this feeling initially by learning more about the individuals and their backgrounds. The information obtained in the application process can be very beneficial to share with the faculty before the class begins. This information may include the participants' educational and experience backgrounds, their responsibilities in their current positions, and their goals in attending this particular course or workshop.

The get-acquainted or warm-up exercise can provide the instructor with more information about the class, including such personal data as interests and hobbies. This helps the learners understand that they are being considered as whole persons, not just a nurse in the Intensive-Coronary Care Unit (ICCU) or Emergency, not just a staff person or supervisor. They find it easier to relate with other persons in the group who share common interests. For example, in the warm-up session for one workshop, the authors found about half the members of the group enjoyed sewing as a hobby but found it difficult to find any time for this activity. They described the patterns and materials they had planned to use that continued to collect in their closets. This common interest helped these individuals develop into a group in which they felt a common bond and were more at ease with each other, resulting in a more open atmosphere.

The teacher also should be a part of the get-acquainted time, sharing interests and hobbies along with the learners. This helps the class relate to the instructor as an open person who is human and is involved in more than teaching or practicing nursing. This opportunity for sharing supports an atmosphere in which people feel accepted and respected as individuals and not categorized just by the fact that they are nurses or supervisors. By having more data about the learners, the teacher can recognize the resources available in the group.

## Outlining the Course

The objectives, content, and methods to be used in achieving objectives prepared by the planning committee are reviewed with the students as a part of the introduction to the course, workshop, or symposium. This is presented as the program developed by the planning committee and the teacher. The learners then are given an opportunity to participate in determining their objectives for the session within its established framework. This provides for relating the predetermined objectives specifically to those of the class.

The size of the group dictates how this can be accomplished. If it is a small group, it may be possible to do this individually or collectively using an idea inventory or brainstorming session. If it is a larger group, it may be necessary to divide the nurses into smaller units with each establishing its objectives. Whichever technique is used, it should be emphasized that the teachers are seeking concepts, not well-stated behavioral objectives. Writing behavorial objectives is not the purpose of this session; the teachers are trying to find out exactly what this group is seeking in terms of learning. The group should not be permitted to spend so much time deciding how to state the objective that it loses the purpose and focus of the exercise. If they wish, teachers have an opportunity to help nurses learn more about stating objectives as the group presents these session goals, but this is not the focus.

Participant or learner objectives should be recorded in such a way that the objectives can be retained and posted throughout the class. If this is being done in smaller groups, with each reporting separately, there probably will be some duplication, which is eliminated in the recording provided the groups agree the meaning is the same.

After all objectives are recorded, the total group works with the instructor in establishing priorities and determining which ones can be attained realistically within the time frame, planned content, and teaching methods. For example, if a two-day workshop on basic cardiac arrhythmias is being conducted and the learners want to be able to identify *all* cardiac dysrhythmic patterns, this is an unrealistic objective for so short a time span. The teacher should discuss this objective in terms of why the nurses set this as an expected outcome and why it is unrealistic.

The opportunity for learners to be involved in setting objectives helps clarify the differences in the perceptions and expectations of the planners, teacher, and nurses themselves. This will help prevent much frustration and dissatisfaction among the students. Closely allied with the intense need for knowledge and skills that can be applied immediately on the job is the urgency to learn a great deal in a short time. By having the nurses provide their objectives, the instructor can help them identify some of their expectations as unrealistic. This must be done in such a way that the students do not feel the teacher is exerting authority or making decisions about objectives arbitrarily. The instructor and learners may reach a consensus that there is a need for planning additional educational activities in order to meet the objectives set by the participants. The alert staff coordinator can use this as the first step in planning additional sessions for this class and establish a planning committee from the group.

## Physiological Environment

Growth and developmental concepts throughout the life cycles are important considerations in adult education. Not only is the psychological environment an important consideration in the learning climate but so too are the physical factors required to make the students comfortable. Persons involved in providing continuing education in nursing and staff development programs need a thorough knowledge of the physiological changes of normal aging and the implications these changes hold for the adult since the continuing education program serves nurses of all ages.

Visual acuity is of concern for all age groups. However, there is a steady decrease in the average efficiency of all measurable visual functions in the aging process, even in otherwise healthy eyes. The educational facility should have good illumination since older adults need not only better light but also more light. The class should not face the light, such as a window, and should be seated close to the speaker and to materials used in demonstrations. If audiovisuals are used, all participants should be seated so that they can see all parts of the screen. Sharp color contrasts on charts, diagrams, or pictures are helpful. There should not be a shiny slateboard that creates a glare and is difficult to read. In preparing materials for duplication, large type should be used, with double-spacing for easy reading.

Not being able to hear what is being discussed is frustrating in any class. Auditory changes do occur in the process of aging. Teachers of adults need to speak more slowly and distinctly. Unusual words, unfamiliar terms, and the like should be put on the slateboard, overhead projector, or newsprint. Both the teacher and the staff should be sensitive to nonverbal communications by studying the nurses' actions and reactions. The expressions on their faces, a demonstrated loss of interest by their position, or other behaviors may indicate they cannot hear. The teacher should face and talk directly to the group. From careful observation, the teacher may find some learners consciously or unconsciously depending on lip-reading. Some persons may not realize any loss of hearing since it is a gradual process, while others do not wish to admit to such a loss. The teacher who makes this observation should stand in the same location with a minor amount of moving around and face the individual as much as possible. Noises inside and outside of the room should be eliminated if possible. If an outside noise is being created by construction or other type of activity that cannot be eliminated, an effort should be made to move to another location.

When a member of the group asks a question, the teacher should repeat it before responding so that everyone will know what is being discussed. The staff person may sit in the rear of the room to call the teacher's attention to instances when the group cannot hear or when materials cannot be seen so the situation can be corrected. Attention should be given to the room's acoustics and the availability of a sound system.

As people become older, they tend to correlate ideas more slowly. Organizing material in a logical sequence with a central focus will assist students to relate better to the learning experience. It also is important to recognize that the speed with which adults accomplish tasks diminishes with age. Lack of swiftness and comprehension should not be equated with loss of intelligence or lack of ability. Adults tend to master what is expected of them when they are given the time necessary to achieve at their own rate.

The furniture used and its arrangement also are important in providing for the physical comfort of the class. Adults may find it difficult to sit in desk chairs provided in many classrooms and may feel they are being treated as children. Where possible, tables and comfortable chairs should be used.

Sitting for long periods of time is as difficult for adults as for young people. Frequent breaks are necessary, especially for nurses who are used to being very active during the work day. Bodily functions may not always be as much under control as they once were so adequate bathrooms must be available. Breaks also provide good opportunities for socialization as the students have an opportunity to become better acquainted with each other and with the faculty.

Adults are less tolerant of uncomfortable surroundings, especially when attending a class voluntarily. Maintaining the temperature at a comfortable level and providing adequate ventilation are crucial.

Physical comfort is extremely important to adults. The staff and the faculty should be sensitive to such needs. Learners who are too cold or too hot, cannot see what is being demonstrated, or cannot hear what is being said not only are uncomfortable but also find learning difficult.

## THE TEACHER OF ADULTS

In approaching the class, the teacher must keep in mind some basic concepts of adult education:

1. Adults have determined their own self-concept and expect to be perceived as self-directing and capable of assuming responsibility for their own lives as well as their own learning. They feel they know who they are, what their capabilities are, and how best to use them. If they find themselves in a situation in which the teacher does not recognize the ability to be self-directing, they can be expected to develop resentment and resistance that will interfere with their ability to learn.
2. Adults have gone through the maturation process during which they have accumulated the variety of experiences that provide a broad base

on which to build new learning. The teacher must recognize and use these experiences. Adults are looking for experiential types of teaching techniques that allow them to be involved. Their experiences also have had a major impact on their self-concept and have been used to define who they are.

3. Adults' readiness to learn in continuing education is related to the problems they are encountering in their everyday life situations. They are beyond the phase of having to enroll in courses under pressure to meet some academic requirement. They are seeking new information and skills that they can use on the job or in their life situation and that will enable them to do a better job.

4. Adults seeking new learning are operating in the here-and-now, not future, application of this information. Adults want learning to be problem centered and immediately applicable. They enter the class seeking solutions to problems they are encountering on the job. They want to gain experience that will allow them to return to their positions and solve problems that had been interfering with their doing good work or institute new techniques that will enable them to perform better.

The teacher of adults, like the learners themselves, enters the educational situation with more than expertise in a certain subject area and the ability to present content. Instructors bring certain concepts about teaching; certain self-concepts; and certain values, beliefs, and ideas. It is to be hoped that their teaching concepts are compatible with what is known about learning transactions in adult education.

Teaching is a human relations activity requiring an understanding of the interactions that take place within a group and of the interpersonal skills that enhance interactions. The teacher's role is to facilitate a relationship with the students that will enable both the class and the individuals to identify the group goals and the relationships that will enhance the learning activity. This is why it is important to provide the introductory phase and objective-setting exercise. This process initiates interactions between the teacher and the learners and among the students themselves. The teacher not only will be able to determine the group's needs but also in the process will uncover some of the needs of its members. The group's goals themselves usually are a composite of those of its members. This enables the teacher to get a feeling for the needs of the individuals.

## Learners As Persons

The teacher must accept the nurses as persons with individual needs, motives, expectations, values, and self-perceptions, all of which have an impact on what happens in class. The get-acquainted session gives some insight into the learners as persons. Throughout the course, the teacher should gain additional insight into the students. The nurses need to sense that the teacher accepts them through demonstrating respect and willingness to listen. There is a two-way sense of a helping relationship. For example, nurses who work in smaller health care facilities may not have the support services, staff, and other elements required to implement specific programs in the same way larger facilities can. An educator teaching a specific program such as developing a patient classification system should listen to the learners, respect the differences that exist, and help them evolve alternative approaches that they might use. The teacher who is unable to relate to the learners' problems and help them cope with these issues will lose their attention as they find themselves frustrated and tense.

The teacher needs skill in class leadership and an understanding of group process. In the leadership role, the instructor is concerned with achieving the established course objectives and at the same time encouraging group growth and interaction. There are a number of development models, such as Tuckman's[8] and Schein's,[9] which describe systematic ways of looking at the stages, sequences, and phases that groups develop. Groups of learners begin as a collection of people who are attending an educational session with some common objectives. The teacher is concerned that this collection of individuals has the opportunity to grow as a group in its ability to deal with its human relations problems and at the same time accomplish the course objectives.

## The Two-Dimensional Approach

To facilitate group growth and at the same time accomplish the objectives, the teacher should have some knowledge of the stages of group development in task functions and personal relations. John E. Jones, a consultant in team development and intergroup relations, describes a two-dimensional approach to groups and their development that can be used by the teacher in continuing education in nursing: (1) personal relations and (2) task functions.[10]

Personal relations are described as the human side of the activity within the group. "Personal relations involves how people feel about each other, how people expect each other to behave, the commitments that people develop to each other, the kind of assumptions that people make about each other, and the kinds of problems that people have in joining forces in order to get the work done."[11] In this situation, the work or task is learning and the teacher must be cognizant of the human relations dimension of the group. Like any other group, the class begins as a collection of individuals who come together with certain expectations and concerns. Initially, the group depends on the teacher to provide structure and direction. It is concerned with orientation to what is going to happen. The teacher should be aware of the initial stage of group development and support the group, realizing that the process takes time.

The teacher assumes a primary role in initiating the other dimension of group development described by Jones—the task function. "A group comes together, learns what the task is, mobilizes to accomplish the task and does the work."[12] The teacher has to achieve a balance between the two dimensions. The educator's concern must be getting the task done but without sacrificing the human relations activity that is essential for the group's growth. Being familiar with the stages of group development enables the teacher to determine the level of functioning of a particular class. This will assist the teacher in diagnosing problems the learners may be having. This knowledge also will help the instructor in determining the timing for particular activities.

## Four Developmental Stages

There are four stages of development that occur in groups organized for a specific activity, such as learning. In the initial phase the group is concerned with orientation to the task. Personal relations functions consist of dependency: the group members expect the teacher to assume the responsibility for what is happening and what is expected of them. They depend on the teacher to be the leader and define the ground rules and structure. The teacher's recognition of this stage of development is a part of the orientation or get-acquainted exercise and objective setting described in the previous section. The instructor realizes at this stage that the class is not ready to assume a major role in the learning activities.

In stage two of group development, the members are concerned with the way to organize to accomplish the task. In using a group assignment at this stage, it will take time for the members to make decisions about how they will go about achieving the assignment—the organizational phase of their task functions. During this phase, conflict or disagreements usually emerge in the human relations functions. The teacher is the facilitator and intervenes in the group activity only when asked to clarify something or when it is obvious the members have reached an impasse that they cannot deal with themselves. If the instructor provides too much assistance, the group will continue to be dependent. This will stifle creativity and delay group growth.

In the third stage, the group has developed to the point that its members feel comfortable with the task and with each other. There is a sense of belonging. The group organizes the way it will proceed to accomplish the task, makes decisions about acceptable behavior (norms), and its members assume roles that are directed at moving it toward achievement of the task and toward maintaining the group process. There is a sharing of ideas, an exploration of actions related to the task, and a good flow of communications.

In the final stage, the group members can function interdependently in the human relations area. They can solve problems posed by the task. The teacher is used only to provide additional information the group may need for achieving the task, which it is highly motivated to accomplish. The members can handle interpersonal relations problems that may occur as they work toward achieving the objective. This is referred to as the stage at which a group can perform.

## Behavior and Development

Throughout the course, the teacher needs to be aware of the behaviors identified with the development of human relations and task dimensions within the group. By observing the way the group is functioning, the educator can intervene at appropriate times to provide feedback on what is happening. Teacher support and encouragement facilitate group growth; however, too much assistance prevents its development. The teacher should be skilled in determining when to intervene and when the group needs feedback.

The teacher serves as a role model for learning. In introducing the educational offering and the approaches to be used to achieve the expected outcome, the emphasis is on the dual role of teacher and learner and on the expectation of gaining new information from the experience. Throughout the course, the teacher demonstrates the role of the learner through active participation in the group and by expressing interest in the ideas and concepts that are being shared and that may provide new insight for the instructor. By displaying openness, by respecting others' ideas or opinions even if different, and by accepting each person as an individual, the teacher serves as a role model for the other learners. A demonstration of the teacher's own experiences serves as a learning resource.

The teacher must communicate effectively, both verbally and nonverbally. Listening is an essential component of the communication process. Adults are encouraged to share ideas and in return expect the teacher to be an effective listener. Learners are sensitive to the teacher's nonverbal communications such as facial expressions and gestures. Some gestures may be distracting, and the teacher needs to be sensitive to the potential effect of those that are used. The teacher should articulate effectively in communicating verbally. Most teachers, as well as other persons, may be unaware of how they sound and of some of the expressions they use, such as "you know" in every other sentence. This may distract the nurses from the subject while they count the number of "you know's" the teacher uses. To increase teachers' awareness of how they sound, audiotapes can be very revealing and provide the impetus for changing the way they communicate verbally. Videotapes also provide cues to nonverbal communications.

Teachers must be fully cognizant of the course content in terms of both the knowledge base and the skills required in its application. Nurse learners expect teachers to present the theoretical base for practice in a particular specialty or area and to apply the theory to the practice arena. This is not to say the instructor must know everything. Learners' practice areas may be very different from those of the teacher. In such a situation, the teacher works to apply the material to the particular practice settings based on the theoretical principles. The teacher does need to display self-confidence but at the same time should be open about a lack of knowledge or about mistakes. If supplemental teaching aids are to be used, the teacher must assume responsibility for their effective use.

Teachers must be able to help individuals or groups in dealing with interpersonal problems that may arise. Counseling skills may be necessary, particularly if the group does not deal with the problem. The individual who has been "sent" to the class may be a case in point. By arranging to talk with that individual during a break, the teacher may be able to uncover some of the person's needs or interests. The attention given by the teacher may be all the person needs to at least be receptive to the course content even if the individual never progresses to the level of active participation. The teacher may be able to assist the individual to determine a relationship between needs or interests and learning.

Numerous problems may occur in group dynamics, particularly in learning experiences that involve a large number of joint activities. Teachers should be familiar with both members' behavior that facilitates the work of the group and self-centered behavior that interferes with the process. Teachers should know how groups function and how to help them deal with behaviors that disrupt their process.

## SUMMARY

Continuing education classes in nursing and staff development programs have broad goals that include "improved nursing care for patients and clients." If these programs are to achieve this goal, the staff and the teachers must plan and conduct educational offerings based on a learning theory that incorporates elements of adult education and group dynamics. The staff and teachers must be sensitive to the physiological and psychological conditions in the learning environment that enhance adult education.

**NOTES**

1. American Nurses' Association, *Continuing Education in Nursing: An Overview* (Kansas City, Mo.: American Nurses' Association, 1979), p. 6.

2. Preston P. LeBreton, ed., *The Assessment and Development of Professionals: Theory and Practice* (Seattle: University of Washington, 1976), p. 3.

3. Ibid., p. 3.

4. Ibid., p. 3.

5. Ibid., pp. 3–4.

6. Cyril O. Houle, "The Nature of Continuing Professional Education," in *Adult Learning: Issues and Innovations,* Robert E. Smith, ed. (DeKalb, Ill.: Northern Illinois University, July 1976), p. 48.

7. John D. Engalls, ed., *A Trainers' Guide to Andragogy,* 2d rev. ed. (Washington, D.C.: U.S. Department of Health, Education, and Welfare, 1973), p. 7.

8. Bruce W. Tuckman, "Developmental Sequence in Small Groups," *Psychological Bulletin* 63, 1965, pp. 384-399.

9. Edgar H. Schein, *Process Consultation: Its Role in Organization Development* (Reading, Mass.: Addison-Wesley Publishing Company, 1969).

10. John E. Jones, "Model of Group Development," *The 1973 Annual Handbook for Group Facilitators* (La Jolla, Cal.: University Associates), p. 128.

11. Ibid., p. 128.

12. Ibid., p. 128.

# Chapter 2

# Organization and Administration of a Continuing Education and Staff Development Program

## ORGANIZATIONAL FRAMEWORK

The continuing education program usually is established as a structural unit of an existing institution or organization, although some programs are set up as corporate bodies or organizations specifically designed to provide or market such material.

This discussion of the organizational framework focuses on continuing education programs in existing organizations or institutions such as colleges, universities, hospitals, facilities for long-term care, or professional organizations.

### The Mission

The mission, or purpose for existence, of the total organization must be reviewed to determine how the continuing education program will, or does, contribute to the entity's goals. The organization's mission may be stated in a number of different documents and sometimes may be difficult to locate as such. However, a review of the articles of incorporation or the bylaws should reveal the statement of purpose. For example, in a college or university, these statements may appear in the bulletin published for prospective students; in a health care facility, a general statement may be found in the employee or patient handbook.

The organization's mission statement is important because it provides a rationale for the continuing education program. For example, if a mission statement calls for "the provision of nondegree programs, courses, and workshops to meet the lifelong learning needs in academic, occupational, professional, cultural, and avocational areas," a university can legitimately support a continuing education program for health professionals as a way to fulfill that objective. A health care facility whose mission includes statements relating to patients' rights to "the highest quality care provided by health care personnel who are aware of the most up-to-date methods of care and treatment" has a responsibility to provide its personnel with opportunities to update their knowledge and skills. The facility must decide whether to establish a continuing education and staff development program or to depend on other similar programs. The important consideration is the facility's responsibility for the education of its employees to fulfill its mission. A professional organization that includes in its statement of purpose "provision of education for members" must determine the structure and financing it will need to achieve this objective.

The mission statement also should be studied to determine the overall goal of the continuing education program. Does the statement limit what the program can do? Can the program address the personal growth needs of health care professionals or must it be limited to the professional knowledge and skills they require to provide patient services? Must it be limited to professional knowledge and skills that can be used in that particular health care facility? Is the program intended to serve only members of the organization or institution or may nonmember professionals attend? Such issues must be addressed and clarified in establishing a continuing education program. The organization or institution's general mission determines the continuing education program's goal, which in turn determines the instructional programming.

## Placement within the Organization

A continuing education program can function under many organizational models, but the operating conditions must be considered carefully before determining its placement in the overall structure. These conditions include:

- What group(s) will the program serve?
- With whom does the program need to have liaison?
- How can the program best influence "improved patient care?"
- How can the program be financed?

In a college or university (Exhibit 2-1), the program placement options usually are in a specific professional school such as nursing, pharmacy, or the school of continuing studies. Some factors to be considered in determining placement are:

**Exhibit 2-1** Organizational Chart—College/University Continuing Education in Nursing Program

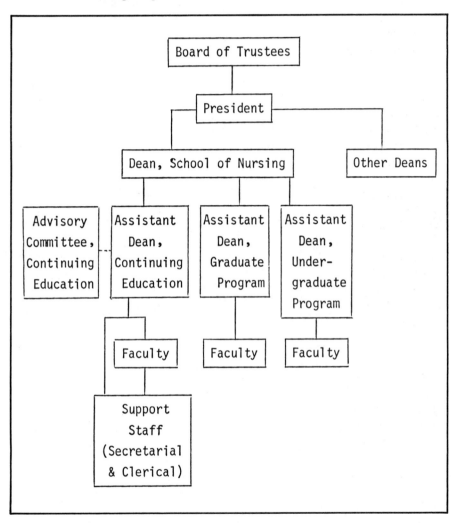

- faculty status for staff in the particular school or department

- support of full-time faculty in other educational programs in the school (such as those in the baccalaureate and graduate departments) in teaching in continuing education

- support services available

- financial support

- clients to be served

- involvement in policy decisions related to continuing education

- requirements of accreditation or approval processes

Dual faculty appointments for the staff may be possible, with the opportunity to have input in, and support from, both the professional school and the continuing education department. Having the resources available to accomplish the program's mission is the prime consideration. Most professions feel this is accomplished best by establishing the program as a unit of the professional school.

In a health care facility, the options are similar. Will each department have a continuing education program specific to the needs of its personnel or will a facilitywide operation for all employees be established? In a facilitywide education department, the instructional program is centralized and all departments collaborate in determining and planning for needs of their personnel. Traditionally, health care facilities have had organized nursing inservice or staff development departments that sometimes cooperated with other units in providing education for nonnursing personnel. As departments and staff have been added, these facilities and their accrediting bodies have recognized the need for education for all personnel, resulting in the establishment of more institutionwide programs.

The facilitywide program has the advantage of centralizing educational resources in one department that can maximize the benefits to the entire institution. A new department may be established to assume responsibility for continuing education or the function may be undertaken by an existing department such as personnel or nursing inservice or staff development. The separate education department has the advantages of having instruction as its main function, maintaining a separate budget, responding to the needs of all personnel, and coordinating all training activities. A major problem for the education department is acquiring the support of all other units in identifying needs and resources and planning instructional programs.

Larger facilities may continue to operate a separate nursing inservice unit, with all other instruction and training handled by the education department.

In many institutions, this has resulted in decentralizing staff development within the nursing department. For example, one member of the staff development department may be responsible for education for the units caring for patients with coronary disease, including intensive care, the "step down" unit (unit for transferring patients who do not need the more intensive care but who continue to need cardiac monitoring), and cardiac rehabilitation.

The professional association may delegate its education responsibility to one of its commissions or committees, with that unit's representative assuming all staff functions for education. A full-time staff member may be required if: (1) education is a major function of the association, (2) continuing education is a requirement for the profession, or (3) an approval/accreditation process requires a separate education unit.

## Primary Service Area

The service area for a continuing education program must be consistent with its mission. A major college or university may view its mission as providing continuing education for health professionals from its own state and from other states, particularly if it has the only professional school in that state for the basic preparation of personnel for specific fields such as pharmacy, physical therapy, or medicine. A regional college or university may view its mission as serving a designated area of its state.

## PHILOSOPHY AND GOALS

A philosophy can be defined as a system of beliefs that directs an organization in achieving its mission or purpose and provides a basis for decision making in defining how the objective is to be accomplished. It should be a "working" philosophy, which means it should *not* be an elaborate statement of concepts or beliefs derived from a review of other philosophies or written in professional jargon. Rather, it should be a statement of the organization's beliefs in determining the approach to be used in achieving its defined mission.

In defining the philosophy of the continuing education department, the beliefs of the organization of which it is a part must be examined. The philosophy of any component must be in accord with that of the organization of which it is a part.

The continuing education department's philosophy should address the values and beliefs that affect the decisions to be made by the administration, staff, and teachers in the instruction to be provided.

In stating the philosophy for a continuing education program for health care professionals, some areas that need to be examined are:

- Beliefs about health care, including individuals' rights to health care
- Beliefs about the contribution or responsibility of health care personnel in providing services
- Beliefs of the organization's responsibility for providing education to assist personnel in improving health care
- Beliefs about the responsibility of individual practitioners for their own continuing education
- Beliefs about learning and how it takes place
- Beliefs about teaching and teaching methods that facilitate learning
- Beliefs about continuing evaluation and improvement of the education program

The development of a philosophy for a continuing education program should be a group, not individual, activity. Each program must identify key persons who should contribute to the statement of philosophy. In a college or university, the department or division staff may prepare the program philosophy for review, discussion, and approval by the institution's faculty. If there is only one staff member in the continuing education department, then a committee of other faculty members may be established to identify the beliefs. The philosophy for continuing education is a part of the total school and therefore must be understood and accepted by the entire faculty (Exhibit 2-2).

In a health care facilitywide continuing education department the staff may initiate the statement of beliefs for presentation to and input from all departments. Since the program is a provider of educational services for all departments, the philosophy must incorporate their beliefs. As with the college or university, the staff may be too small and a committee of representatives of all departments may have to develop and review the philosophy. Final approval is by the administration or board. The same process is applicable for nursing's inservice or staff development program when it is a separate and distinct unit and responsible only for that department (Exhibit 2-3).

The professional association usually depends upon the organized unit assigned the responsibility for the continuing education of its members to initiate the statements of beliefs. This may be a committee, council, or commission that will draft the statement for review and acceptance by the association's board or ultimate authority group.

In developing the philosophy for a continuing education in nursing program, the guidelines established by the accrediting body should be followed.

**Exhibit 2-2** Example of a Philosophy Statement

---

### INDIANA UNIVERSITY SCHOOL OF NURSING
### CONTINUING EDUCATION PROGRAM
### PHILOSOPHY

Nursing is a service involving a collaborative relationship among nurses, clients/patients and other members of the health care team for the purposes of health maintenance, restoration and reorganization through the use of the nursing process. The goal of nursing is to assist individuals to achieve cooperatively determined health goals and to reach a level of adaptation consistent with their unique health-illness state. Nursing practice is derived from a knowledge of the principles of biological, physical and behavioral sciences and through the use of research findings. This practice is characterized by dependent, independent, and interdependent nursing actions leading to quality health care.

We believe that nursing has as its primary concern the welfare of human beings as prescribed by the highly complex and changing needs of society. The dynamic nature of society demands that nursing education be flexible in order to adapt to the continuing process of these changing needs.

We believe that consumers of health care are demanding and will continue to demand an increasing degree of accountability for nursing competence. Continuing education is one mechanism of providing for the upgrading of knowledge and skills for the maintenance of nursing competence. The concept of continuing education begins in an initial nursing education program. The motivation and responsibility for continued competency rests with the individual nurse throughout the nursing career. The extent to which individual nurses assume this responsibility is influenced by a synthesis of external factors, intellectual curiosity, analytical thinking, and creativity in working with and through others in the delivery of optimal health care. The Indiana University School of Nursing Continuing Education Program is concerned with continued learning for nurses which will increase competence and enhance their ability to influence the direction of optimal health care delivery.

We believe that adults are problem-oriented, self directed, and possess varied competencies as a result of their life experiences. Therefore, the approach to adult learning involves cooperative teacher-learner interaction in the application of knowledge and the evaluation of progress toward the achievement of the learner's goals.

We accept the responsibility of a role model for teaching, research, and public service for continued growth and development toward excellence in nursing practice. We perceive our primary responsibility to be the provision of oppor-

---

**Exhibit 2-2** continued

tunities through which nurses may increase their knowledge and skills on a continuum throughout their careers. This responsibility includes the collaboration between university faculty and health care agency personnel; the provision of offerings predicated on the capabilities and needs of the nurse and on the emerging patterns of health care delivery; and the provision of an educational environment conducive to the learner's self-direction, self-inquiry, and self-actualization.

*Source:* Continuing Education Program, Indiana University School of Nursing, Indianapolis, Indiana. Reprinted with permission, 1980.

---

For example, the American Nurses' Association's *Accreditation of Continuing Education in Nursing* states:

1. The philosophy, purpose, and goals of the agency or organization indicate a concern for the promotion and advancement of health care and continuing education in nursing.
2. The philosophy contains a statement of belief about the nature of nursing and continuing education in that field.
3. The philosophy, purpose, and goals of the provider unit are consistent with those of the agency or organization.
4. The philosophy, purpose, and goals show evidence of review within the last four years and are up-to-date.

The philosophy for the continuing education program in any of the organizations should be stated in terms that are understood and can be used by all persons involved in its implementation. The statement of philosophy is not a static array of words but rather a "working" set of beliefs that is used, is reexamined periodically to be sure it still serves its purpose, and is changed in accordance with developments in the mission or purpose.

The goals of the continuing education program evolve from the mission (purpose) and the philosophy. Goals are broad statements of what the program expects to accomplish, from which action-oriented short-range and long-range objectives may be defined. The objectives are written in terms of results expected, which then can be used in evaluating program achievements.

The relationship of the purpose, philosophy, and goals is demonstrated by excerpts from sample statements of each (Exhibit 2-4).

**Exhibit 2-3** Example of a Staff Development Statement

---

### REID MEMORIAL HOSPITAL

#### Definition of Staff Development

A method of informal education by which an employee may be developed to fulfill specific job duties/responsibilities. Such a method includes varying teaching/learning techniques (i.e.: didactic, clinical experience, workshops, conferences) and is influenced by the involvement of all persons responsible for employee activity. Staff development begins with orientation and is continued through in-service programs and continuing education activities.

#### Philosophy

We of the department of staff development, Reid Memorial Hospital, believe:

That each patient is entitled to receive effective, efficient, considerate and safe care.

That such care can only be provided by employees who have the necessary knowledge, skills and attitudes.

That the individual employee must be developed in accordance with the desirable standards of the employer in order to develop competence that will be reflected in both quantity and quality of nursing care.

That there must be continual staff development for all personnel. The programs offered are to be planned for the level and scope of individual groups, and to their defined duties/responsibilities.

That such development should begin with employment and end only with termination from employment, providing appropriate orientation and continuous opportunities for learning which will enable the employee to function and develop to his job level.

That programs should be initiated to meet the expressed needs of specific departments. That Staff Development Department should assist in defining these needs through participating in research under direction of department involved.

That continuing education is separate and distinct from On-The-Job training and/or In-Service.

That Continuing Education is necessary in order to promote the growth and development of employees and to support the concept of upward mobility in careers and life-long learning.

That Continuing Education is an integral part of the change process. It provides opportunity for the health care professional to actively prepare for and respond to change.

That continuing education program development should be based on accepted adult education principles.

**Exhibit 2-3** continued

That the American Nurses' Association's and Indiana State Nurses' Association's standards for the approval of continuing education programs and offerings for nursing are appropriate and should be utilized.

That Continuing Education sponsored by Staff Development should provide a positive influence on health care practitioners and on health care practice, providing information about forces for change, approaches for responding to change and skills necessary to initiate change.

That content of Staff Development Orientation, On-The-Job training, and In-Service programs should reflect the employer's current philosophies, policies, and procedures.

That intra and inter departmental cooperation is necessary for successful employee development.

That individuals interested in enlarging their field of knowledge and expertise should be supported through programs of financial assistance made available through assigned department and/or Personnel.

*Source:* Reprinted from *Operations Manual*, Department of Staff Development, Reid Memorial Hospital, Richmond, Indiana, by permission of Doris S. Mettert, Director, ©1980.

## STAFFING

### Administrative

The administrator of a continuing education program, like any other executive, must possess a number of characteristics in order to be successful: a high degree of administrative skill and thorough knowledge of continuing education program planning, adult education, budgeting, and management.

Continuing educators enter the field from a variety of backgrounds because it has no shared educational or experiential basis, as do many other disciplines. Therefore, the education director must be aware of the scope of the field, the issues (both current and emerging), and trends.

The program director also must be familiar with organizational theory. The parent organization within which the program functions is a major source of influence on its operations, so the director needs a basic operational knowledge of how organizations work and, more importantly, how to influence them. Most organizations with these programs have missions other than continuing education as their primary focus. Therefore, the director must understand the total purpose of the institution and how the program fits into

**Exhibit 2-4** Sample Statements

---

**PURPOSE**

The Continuing Education in Nursing Program has as its purpose to provide noncredit continuing education in nursing offerings for registered nurses in (area-location) based on the needs of the individuals and the changing patterns of health care delivery that impact on nursing care.

**PHILOSOPHY**

We believe professional continuing education in nursing consists of a variety of planned learning experiences beyond the basic nursing educational program that are designed to enhance nursing practice by expanding the nurse's knowledge, skills, and attitudes. The planned learning experiences are built upon adult education principles, are specific to the learner's needs, and are immediately applicable to the learner's goal.

**GOAL**

To develop sound educational offerings to meet the identified needs of nurses in the (region, area, state, hospital).

---

that framework. Educational exposure to organizational behavior as well as experience in institutions, particularly in administrative roles, is a prerequisite for a successful director.

The program director must be thoroughly conversant with the program planning process—several models are available (Chapter 4) and may be used at various times. The director generally will be assisting others as they learn the planning process and so must be experienced in how to apply it.

The program director must be knowledgeable about adult education and the physiology and psychology of adulthood if the courses are to be relevant to their target groups.

*The Effective Practitioner*

The continuing educator who incorporates the characteristics of knowledge of the field, the program planning process, and understanding of adult development and learning generally will be an effective practitioner. The administrator also must be proficient in budgeting and managing.

The skill needed for budgeting may be limited to calculating costs for specific educational activities and determining the appropriate registration fees, paying the bills, and finally striking a balance of overage or deficit. Or the budgeting process may be more complex, with the program director having full fiscal control over an entire department. The skills required for each of these two situations vary widely. The director who does not possess these skills can turn for help to the many continuing education activities in attempting to acquire the necessary mastery.

The continuing education administrator must work with many diverse groups. Within the department, the director has the responsibility of managing a staff that may include other professional continuing educators and support personnel of various kinds, depending on the size of the organization. The successful administrator uses the varying talents and capabilities of these individuals to the greatest extent, capitalizing on their strengths and minimizing their weaknesses.

The responsibility of both failures and successes in the department is shared. Everyone involved must understand how the department functions within the institution and demonstrate a commitment to the entire organization and its goals as well as to the program and its objectives. The need for the administrator to be an emotionally and professionally mature person cannot be overemphasized.

The administrator should be prepared both academically and experientially for the position. Academic preparation should include exposure to adult education, organizational behavior, research, and evaluation. The director of a continuing education program in nursing should be a nurse, with clinical, educational, and administrative experience in that discipline.

### Personal Characteristics

Personal characteristics of the director are similar to those required for faculty in continuing education (Chapter 7), particularly if the individual is to be involved in teaching in addition to the administrative responsibilities.

The administrator must demonstrate a commitment to lifelong learning. Serving as a role model for faculty and staff is part of the responsibility. The director demonstrates this commitment through knowledge of the field, participation in continuing education offerings, reading professional journals, involvement such as membership in professional organizations, serving on committees, and in elected or appointed positions, research and evaluation activities, and publications. If the director is committed to continuing education, that enthusiasm for learning will be contagious and evoke similar responses in the staff and faculty. If the administrator also teaches, the students will benefit.

The administrator must be effective in interpersonal communications and, because of the need to deal with such diverse groups, must be able to accept them as they are and help them grow. Effective relationships with a variety of individuals and groups is the basis for a successful education program. The director is sensitive to the needs and interests of others and places these above the fulfillment of any personal needs. Given the concurrent duties of supervision, delegation, coordination, staffing, and acquisition of resources, the administrator must have the ability to use persuasion and compromise to foster a climate of cooperation instead of competition, both inside and outside the institution. This cannot be overemphasized as a crucial characteristic.

The administrator must be flexible, innovative, and creative. Because the organization focuses on aspects other than continuing education, the administrator must deal with multiple priorities and programs and with allocation of resources that may be less than those necessary for operation of the program. Competition from other local continuing education programs requires the ability to plan effectively and creatively.

The continuing educator who is learning continuously can acquire characteristics that the individual did not possess when entering the field either in an educational environment (formal or informal) or through experience.

## Professional Staff

The administrator should use care in selecting professional staff members to work in the planning, implementing, and evaluating of continuing education activities (Chapter 7). The administrator should attempt to choose those who will contribute the most to the program's overall mission, and in turn the staff members must accept the responsibilities inherent in involvement with such a department—both for teaching and for routine tasks. Committee assignments are an integral responsibility of professional staff. Staff members with faculty appointments in a college or university may chafe at the necessity for attending faculty meetings, feeling that their time could be spent better in planning courses. The administrator must strike a balance between the staff's responsibility to the institution as a whole and to the continuing education department. Professional staff members are expected to follow the organization's policies and procedures; it is the administrator's responsibility to interpret them and to monitor adherence.

A staff works best in an environment that is conducive to innovation and personal growth. The administrator has the responsibility to provide that environment, to create opportunities for staff members in which they may attain their potential, and to encourage continuing learning. The administrator also must supervise and appraise the performance of all staff members in the education department.

## Support Staff

A support staff, adequate in number and in qualifications, is essential for operation of a continuing education program. The secretarial staff must have basic skills such as typing, shorthand, and filing. Those in contact with the public—answering telephone inquiries, registering participants, and so on—must have good interpersonal skills. Public relations is an essential component of an effective program. Since much of its effectiveness depends on the cooperation of others, support persons who lack the ability to present the program well to the public have no place in the public eye. Other support persons may be available to the department but not be part of the physical staffing pattern. These include computer personnel or those from audiovisual departments.

## Job Descriptions

Each person in the continuing education department should have a well-written job description. It should include the educational and experiential qualifications for the position and a detailed set of performance expectations. Where possible, these job descriptions should be written with input from the incumbents since they know better than anyone what their job requires and what their responsibilities entail. These job descriptions should be used as the basis of the performance appraisal conducted regularly by the department supervisors. The descriptions should be revised whenever there are changes in the jobs.

## ADVISORY COMMITTEES

An advisory committee for continuing education programs can be a valuable asset. It can be useful in the identification of educational needs and of potential resources. It can serve a wide range of purposes, depending on the program's philosophy, goals, and mission. It provides a mechanism for a wide range of involvement, including using the talents and expertise of its members in program planning.

The advisory committee is included in the department's organizational structure. Its relationship is defined clearly on the organizational chart and in the statements of purposes and functions. The committee serves to provide advice to the program and not to make decisions.

In developing an advisory committee, the department first must propose an organizational structure including purposes, functions, and suggested membership categories, plus a meeting schedule. This proposal should be presented to the appropriate individual or group for approval. In a college or university, the dean of the school may approve; for the staff development department, the director of nursing may provide the approval; in a professional association, the decision may require acceptance by a commission or the board. The decision on who must approve may be related to the budgetary implications if members are to be paid for their services or travel for meetings. In most situations the advisory committee members donate their time and may assume travel costs.

The committee membership usually is defined according to the type of representation desired to accomplish the group's purposes. This decision also is based on the program mission, which defines the target audience in both nursing practice and geographical areas. A program organized to serve the total state and nurses in all types of practice should have representatives from all areas of the state and of nursing. Committee members in a program designed to serve a region of the state and specific types of nursing practice should be representative of that region and target audience. A staff development program that serves only the nurses in the facility should include all the fields of practice represented. The professional association serves all its members and will determine representation both geographically and in terms of their specialty categories.

Another membership consideration is the type of expertise needed. This could be provided by persons drawn from voluntary health organizations, health planning agencies, adult and continuing education programs, administration of health care facilities, etc. Representatives of other health professions may be included to strengthen collaboration with these groups.

The decision on who will be chosen may rest with the program staff or with the person or group that approves the establishment of the committee. Staff members definitely should have input into the selection of advisory committee individuals because they tend to have more knowledge of prospective choices and how their capabilities match those needed to achieve the group's purpose.

The persons selected should be invited by letter. To help them decide whether they are to serve, the letter should outline the proposed purposes, functions, and meeting schedules, whether they will be paid or are expected to donate their time, and who will be responsible for the cost of attending meetings.

The first meeting of the advisory committee is planned by the staff and chaired by a staff person. The purposes, functions, and schedule for meetings are reviewed and agreed on. The committee decides on its organizational structure and procedures and elects its officers. A staff person may serve as the recorder of minutes. For future meetings, whoever chairs the committee works with the professional staff in preparing the agenda.

The amount of organizational structure and the number of meetings will depend on the committee's functions. The group may be used in gathering data about educational needs and assisting the staff in establishing priorities for programming. It may help the staff in evaluating the program to determine progress toward its goals. It may work on the development of broad operating policies. The committee members serve as communication links to interpret the programs to the area or group they represent. They can be useful in marketing the program.

Success in using an advisory committee is based on making proper choices of representatives and then keeping its members apprised of the program activities. They need to feel that their involvement is contributing to the success of the program and that the staff perceives that their advice is valuable.


## BUDGETS FOR CONTINUING EDUCATION

### Operational and Capital Budgets

The department director is responsible for preparing and implementing the departmental budget with input from the staff. The submission and approval process may vary according to the organization, with the final adoption of the total budget for all departments being given by the board. Budgets are prepared for the fiscal year, which varies from organization to organization.

Before beginning to prepare the budget, the staff must agree on goals and plans for the coming year to determine the financial support required to achieve the objectives. The budget translates the department's plans into its financial requirements. It is a guide to be followed by all staff members to contain the cost of operating the continuing education department. It also provides essential financial data for evaluating the program, and it promotes operational efficiency in departmental decision making.

### Two Types to Be Submitted

Departments usually are required to submit two types of budgets or to distinguish between operational and capital requirements. The operational budget defines the department's salary requirements, expendable supplies (those with a short usable life) and related expenses, and travel. The capital budget identifies expenditures for equipment, such as audiovisual gear; furniture, such as classroom tables, chairs, desks, etc.; and renovation that may be needed in the space allocated for continuing education. Some organizations review capital budgets in terms of the institution's total capital needs and prioritize them on an overall rather than departmental basis. The funds available for capital expenditures generally are less than those for operations, so the overall allocations must be made according to the priority of needs to support the plans of the total institution. The continuing education department should give careful consideration to capital requests and be able to justify those expenditures if they are to be viewed as high-priority items. For example, if video equipment is not available, the department staff should explain how it will be used and how it will help implement the continuing education goals.

The preparation of the operational budget starts with review of past budgets and expenditures to determine required changes. If the department is new or has not had a separate budget, the director will need to work closely with the organization's financial or business staff in projecting expenditures based on plans for the year.

Operational budget elements vary according to the expense categories established within an organization. The director must be aware of these categories and prepare the budget accordingly. Several months before new budgets are to be submitted, the department staff reviews the past year's budget in terms of accomplishments and of goals and changes for the next year. From this review the department's operational budget is developed.

*Position and Salary Items*

The personnel budget should include a line item figure for each position, including projected salary and fringe benefits. If the proposed salary includes an increase, then a justification with accompanying evaluation data should be included. If merit increases are awarded on an anniversary date of employment, this information needs to be included. For example, if a staff person is to receive a salary increase in September and the budget begins in July, the line item for that position must include the current payment from July to September plus the percent of increase from September through June to show the total for the position. Fringe benefits usually are projected on a percentage of the base salary, so they also will have to be increased. If salary increases are to be given across the board, the department director needs to be informed of this before preparing the budget.

If a new position is being proposed, it should be included in the budget along with a justification and job description. The justification should include why the position is required in terms of the department's goals and the institution's expectations.

In some budgets, personnel requirements include a category for all salaried positions, professional and clerical, and a separate category for wages or part-time clericals used during peak work periods. In budgeting for the wage category, the staff needs to determine the projected number of hours these persons may be required and their hourly rate of pay.

If the operating budget is to support the continuing education offerings as well as all other departmental activities, the expense for instructors also may be included under the personnel budget, or the organization may prefer to place those individuals under a separate category. If they are under the personnel budget, they usually are listed as part-time instructors to conduct specific classes for a total dollar amount. They usually do not receive fringe benefits, with the possible exception of full-time university faculty employed on an overload basis to teach in continuing education. The department must be aware of the university's policies in using these faculty members.

## Supplies and Expenses

The supplies and expenses budget includes expendable items such as:

- office supplies—paper, pencils, pens, paper clips, staples, etc.
- instructional materials—audiotapes, videotapes, transparencies, film rentals, film purchases, books, copies of articles or pamphlets to be used as handout materials
- printing—photocopying, offset printing of materials (in-house or outside vendor)

The expense category includes other operational costs such as:

- promotion—advertisements, brochure preparation
- rentals—equipment, space
- telephone—long-distance telephone calls
- mailing—bulk mailings (including mailing permit if not paid for by the organization), postage

## Budgeting for Travel

The travel budget should project all anticipated staff and instructor trips pertaining to continuing education offerings that are supported by the operating budget. The travel budget includes staff trips to conduct classes in locations other than the immediate setting (university or college, hospital or long-term care facility, or professional association). Costs of staff participation in conferences and meetings should include registration fees, lodging, meals, transportation, and other miscellaneous items. Travel costs are projected on the basis of the reimbursement guidelines established for the agency or organization in terms of amount paid per mile, the maximum allowed for meals, lodging, and other expenses. Staff members should be aware of the requirements for receipts in order to be reimbursed. They will need to identify the specific conferences, workshops, or meetings most relevant to their functions in order to justify the travel expenditures.

Although the exact content of all such sessions or conferences may not be known, there are specific national and state annual meetings related to the functions of the continuing education staff such as the Society for Hospital Education and Training, Adult Education Association, American Nurses' Association's Council on Continuing Education, and National University Extension Association. Staff members who belong to a specific professional organization need to have the opportunity to attend its meetings to keep abreast of changes in the specialty field. Having travel for meetings and conferences approved in the operating budget facilitates advance planning by the staff.

Other special one-time costs may be placed in a separate category or in the supplies and expenses budget. For example, if the department is seeking separate approval or accreditation for the continuing education program, the expenses related to filing the application plus a site visit (if this is a part of the procedure) should be identified in the budget. Approval of individual activities by a particular professional or approval agency may be included as a part of the instructional expense or in a separate category.

In summary, an operating budget and a capital budget should be prepared and implemented by the continuing education staff. By involving the staff in budget preparation, the department can:

1. project the goals and plans for the year
2. be more aware of the fiscal operation and the importance of providing cost-effective continuing education
3. be prepared to establish priorities if the requested funds are reduced and budget revisions are required.

Budget reductions require reviewing the goals and plans to determine which programming will be changed. The cuts are accommodated more easily if priorities have been established already.

## Budgets for Educational Activities

Each separate educational activity should have a budget that identifies its estimated cost—and estimated income, if applicable. When the activity is supported by the overall departmental budget, only the estimated expenses are required to allocate resources. For example, if the department plans to conduct 10 in-house educational courses in the budget year, the estimated cost of each must be available before the operational budget is prepared and submitted. By establishing the estimated cost of each activity and prioritizing these items, the staff can determine the allocation of the resources available in the approved budget.

Many continuing education activities must be self-supporting, requiring the staff to estimate the total expenses of the courses and to set fees that will provide income sufficient to cover out-of-pocket costs. When all or part of the staff also is supported through income from courses, the time its members devote to planning, conducting, and evaluating the activity must be built into the budget.

## The Basic Breakdown

A budget for a continuing education project should include the following estimated cost items:

- instructor(s)—fees to be paid, as well as travel, including meals, hotel, and other expenses
- coordination—staff travel including meals, hotel, and other expenses
- supplies—folders, certificates, name tags, articles, pamphlets, books, pencils, and paper
- postage—mailings to prospective registrants, to instructors, and to the planning committee
- promotion—preparation and printing of brochures, paid advertising
- space—rental fee for meeting facility
- duplicating—materials to be reproduced for the course such as evaluation forms and handouts
- meals and coffee for participants

If personnel costs (departmental staff time) are to be charged to the educational activity, an estimate of members' and secretaries' time that will be involved is included. A specific formula may exist already for determining this expense or the department may be required to establish a method for identifying the cost of personnel time. For example, a study of the time required for the professional staff member to meet with the planning committee, prepare the budget, make contacts with potential resource persons, arrange for facilities, prepare materials, and other activities must be made. The time devoted to coordinating and implementing the educational activity should be determined, as well as the time afterward for preparing the evaluation summary, communicating with instructor(s), and settling expenditures.

Secretarial costs may be determined in the same way as those of the professional staff by an analysis of the time devoted to each activity in planning, implementing, and summarizing the course. By having the secretary record the amount of time required for specific assignments and determining the average from several courses, an average can be reached for calculating the percentage of the secretary's time devoted to each activity. For example, if the average time required to type each certificate of attendance is three minutes, secretarial time for that function for an anticipated enrollment of 30 would be 90 minutes, which can be translated into a dollar figure based on the amount the secretary is paid per hour.

This time analysis will enable the continuing education department to establish a system or formula for projecting the actual costs of a course. This information is needed in determining the department's actual or real costs even if all staff and secretarial staff positions are budgeted line items.

## Percentages and Point Systems

Some organizations have established percentages or point systems for calculating administrative or staff costs. A percentage of the total specific outlays or out-of-pocket expenses may be used to establish the administrative costs. For example, if the total for instruction, supplies, travel, and other expenses is $700 and the administrative expense has been established at 25 percent, then the total cost is $875 and the fee to be charged to participants is based on that figure.

The department should establish some system for identifying costs for a specific activity. Each course may have an identification number that is used in the budget and on all requisitions for purchasing, printing, and other items that are to be charged to that particular event. The number system may begin with the year; for example, 8001 would be continuing education offering No. 1 for fiscal year 1980. It is important that both the education staff and the accounting department be familiar with whatever system is used.

The fees to be charged participants may be determined on the basis of the total cost of conducting the course divided by the number of anticipated enrollments. In situations where all costs—specific expenses plus administrative outlays—must be covered by the income from enrollments, the fee is based on projected participation. For example, the facility may be able to accommodate 40 persons for the course; however, to be able to conduct the offering without a loss if fewer than 40 enroll, the fee may be based on 30 participants. Another approach may be to review costs that fluctuate with enrollment and establish separate fees for these. For example, if meals are included in the fee cost, this expense will decrease with lower enrollment.

A cost analysis may be used to establish a set fee for education courses based on the number of contact hours or days. This is possible when a department has maintained good financial records over time and has had sufficient experience to determine the average cost per class per contact hour or per day. For example, if the average cost for conducting a course has been determined to be $5 per contact hour, then the fee to participants is the number of contact hours × 5. If the cost has been determined to average $20 per day, the fee is established by multiplying the number of days by 20. This system gives the staff flexibility in establishing minimum enrollments since the costs of some classes can be balanced out with the total income from courses over the full fiscal year rather than from each one individually.

In summary, the staff should budget for and identify expenses related to each offering (Exhibits 2-5 and 2-6) in order to develop historical financial data for future reference and determine the actual costs of continuing education.

## RECORDKEEPING AND REPORTS

Determining what data are needed, and designing a system for compiling and maintaining them, is an essential function of the continuing education staff. In addition to budget and expenditure reports, records need to be maintained for each educational activity and for each participant.

The activities of the staff also should be recorded for use in compiling reports for the department. The content of reports may vary according to the needs of the sponsoring agency or organization but all departments should be required to submit some type of monthly or annual report.

A system of maintaining records for each course should be planned in advance. This system will be revised as the staff gains more experience and as the information changes. The questions to be addressed in determining information requirements for an educational program are:

- What information does the staff need in planning the activity?

- What information is needed in preparing reports on courses?

- What information may be needed for accreditation visits?

- What information do participants need to gain recognition for attendance?

- What information is needed for preparing program reports?

- What other information may be needed later?

**Exhibit 2-5** Example of an Activity Budget

```
                           ACTIVITY BUDGET
ORIGINAL___           DIVISION OF CONTINUING STUDIES      ACTIVITY # _____
REVISED ___             COLUMBUS CAMPUS OF IUPUI          ACCOUNT # _____


   ACTIVITY _____

   SCHEDULED AT _____ FROM _____ 19___ TO_____ 19___

   DAYS _____ HOURS_____ OMIT(DATES)_____

   REGISTRATION TIME AND PLACE _____ COORDINATOR_____
                                                    INSTRUCTOR(S):
   SPONSORING SCHOOL/DEPARTMENT _____
```

| EXPENSE | BUDGET | ACTUAL | | | BUDGET | ACTUAL |
|---|---|---|---|---|---|---|
| 1. INSTRUCTIONAL FEE | ___ | ___ | 14. | INDIVIDUAL FEE ASSESSMENTS___ | | ___ |
| 2. INSTRUCTOR TRAVEL | ___ | ___ | | A._____ @ $_____ | | |
| 3. SUPPLIES | ___ | ___ | | B._____ @ $_____ | | |
| 4. POSTAGE | ___ | ___ | 15. | PAYMENT BY OUTSIDE SPONSOR___ | | ___ |
| 5. ADVERTISING | ___ | ___ | 16. | BY TRANSFER FROM OTHER UNIVERSITY SOURCE | ___ | ___ |
| 6. PROMOTION | ___ | ___ | 17. | OTHER (EXPLAIN) | ___ | ___ |
| 7. DUPLICATING | ___ | ___ | 18. | TOTAL INCOME | ___ | ___ |
| 8. MEALS | ___ | ___ | 19. | BALANCE (18-13) | ___ | ___ |
| 9. COFFEE | ___ | ___ | | REMARKS AND EXPLANATIONS | | |
| 10. OTHER (EXPLAIN) | ___ | ___ | | | | |

```
                                             _____
                                             SUBMITTED BY

                                             _____
                                             REVIEWED:  ASST. DIR. CONT. STUDIES
11. TOTAL SPECIFIC EXPENSE  ___  ___
                                             REVIEWED:  ASST. DIR. BUS. AFFAIRS
12. ADMINISTRATIVE EXPENSE  ___  ___
                                             APPROVED:  DIR. COLUMBUS CAMPUS
13. TOTAL EXPENSES          ___  ___
```

COPIES:  BUSINESS OFFICE (WHITE/BLUE)     DEPARTMENT:  (GREEN/YELLOW)
89

*Source:* Reprinted from *Departmental Operating Manual,* Division of Continuing Studies, Columbus Campus, Indiana University-Purdue University at Indianapolis, ©1980.

**Exhibit 2-6** Example of a Budget Form

INDIANA STATE NURSES' ASSOCIATION

Educational Offering Budget Form

Title of Offering _____

Sponsoring Group _____

Date _____

| | Planned Cost | Actual Cost |
|---|---|---|
| Food: | | |
| Lunch | | |
| Coffee | | |
| Cokes | | |
| Other | | |
| | Total | Total |
| | | |
| Supplies: | | |
| Stencils | | |
| Name Tags | | |
| ISNA Postage | | |
| ISNA Envelopes | | |
| Other Postage | | |
| Other Envelopes | | |
| Paper and Printing: | | |
| fliers | | |
| programs | | |
| handouts | | |
| | Total | Total |
| | | |
| Speakers: | | |
| Fees | | |
| Meals | | |
| Travel | | |
| Lodging | | |
| Other | | |
| | Total | Total |
| | | |
| Staff: | | |
| Meals | | |
| Travel | | |
| Other | | |
| | Total | Total |

**Exhibit 2-6** continued

|  | Planned Cost | Actual Cost |
|---|---|---|
| Planning Committee:<br>  Registration Fees<br>  Other | | |
| CEU Application:<br>  Fee<br>  Printing | | |
|  | Subtotal | Subtotal |
| Administrative Cost (25%)<br>  excluding meals | | |
|  | Grand Total | Grand Total |

Minimum number of participants ____
Registration fees:
  ISNA Member
  Nonmember

BEP:ms

*Source:* Reprinted with permission from Indiana State Nurses' Association Council on Continuing Education, ©1979.

The records (files) for educational events can be divided into active and inactive (those being planned and those completed). The file for courses projected or in process should contain all completed forms or documented evidence of planning and of arrangements made for conducting the classes. This information includes:

- names and addresses of planning committee members
- planning committee minutes
- budget
- letters of faculty appointments or agreements
- curriculum vitae for all faculty members
- letters of arrangements for use of facilities outside of the college, university, or hospital, or reservation of space if being conducted in the institution
- arrangements for meals and refreshments, including signed agreement for costs
- outline for the educational activity
- handout or other materials to be duplicated
- the brochure
- copies of orders submitted for supplies or books
- a copy of the participant evaluation form to be used
- correspondence related to the event
- a copy of the Continuing Education Unit (CEU) approval application (if applicable)
- a copy of the CEU record or certificate to be awarded
- other material related to the course

To reduce the amount of material in the file, a notebook may be established for programs being planned or in progress that contains all financial documentation related to a specific course. Using the number established for each course, a tab is prepared to divide the notebook by classes. All documents related to budget and facility agreements are included.

The secretary checklist (Chapter 8) is included at the beginning of the section for each program. This provides a quick reference for the staff and the secretary in seeking information about a particular course.

## The Essential Materials

When a course is completed, the file is reviewed and nonessential materials deleted. Essential material to be maintained on each program includes:

- the budget and expenditure reports
- the faculty letter of agreement and vitae
- the outline of the activity
- a copy of the brochure
- a summary of the evaluation completed by the participants
- a copy of the certificates or CEU record
- planning committee minutes
- the roster of participants

More detailed information used for the course may be retained for future reference. A separate file may be established for handout materials used in various programs, either by course or by subject area.

Participant records and CEU records (Exhibit 2-7) or certificates of attendance may be filed by class in the course file or by individual. It is essential that the system for participant records provide easy retrieval. Computerized registration systems may be available, particularly in a college or university. Computer systems programmed specifically for continuing education registration enable the department to obtain more information about the participants with greater ease than can be tabulated manually. For example, the staff may wish to know the average age of attenders, the educational level, or the county of residence to determine what population group is being served. This information is difficult to record manually for all participants but can be obtained more easily through a computer system. The participant also benefits from the potential of obtaining a complete transcript of all continuing education events attended at a college, university, or total university complex if the system is designed for a multicampus institution.

The continuing education staff should anticipate requests for verification of attendance from participants or their employers. This makes it essential to establish a system for easy access to attendance records.

## Reporting on a Program

Reports on the program are prepared in accordance with the policies and guidelines established by the agency (university or health care facility) and

**Exhibit 2-7** Example of Continuing Education Record

INDIANA
  STATE
    NURSES'
      ASSOCIATION

2915 North High School Road   •   Indianapolis, Indiana 46224   •   317-299-4575

**CONTINUING EDUCATION UNIT (CEU) RECORD**

DATE_____

I.  PARTICIPANT INFORMATION

NAME_____ SS#(optional) _____
      (last)      (first)      (initial)    (maiden)

HOME ADDRESS _____
              (street)        (city)        (state)      (zip)

LICENSE#_____STATE_____RN_____

R _____

PLACE OF EMPLOYMENT_____

EMPLOYMENT ADDRESS _____
                   (street)       (city)       (state)      (zip)

II.  EDUCATIONAL OFFERING INFORMATION

EDUCATIONAL OFFERING NUMBER_____

TITLE _____

STARTING AND ENDING DATES _____

LOCATION OF OFFERING _____
                (place)       (city)       (state)

PRIMARY SPONSORING AGENCY_____

OFFERING DIRECTOR _____

NUMBER OF CONTACT HOURS  THEORY_____TOTAL_____NUMBER OF CEU _____

                        CLINICAL_____

SIGNATURE_____
                Offering Director

The Indiana State Nurses' Association has been accredited as a provider of continuing education for nursing, by the Central Regional Accrediting Committee of the American Nurses' Association for a period of four years (from March 19, 1980 to March 18, 1984).

ISNA recommends that these CEU Record forms be kept for at least a three (3) year period of time by individuals.

96

9/80                         ◆49

*Source:* ISNA Council on C.E., ©1980.

organization. Reports should include attendance, the number of contact hours, and the number of CEU records or certificates awarded. Reports at colleges or universities usually are compiled on a quarter or semester basis, with the annual report at the end of the academic year. Reports in health care facilities or professional organizations may be prepared more frequently (monthly) in accordance with administrative or board requirements. The education staff in the hospital or long-term care facility may have the additional responsibility of maintaining records of all staff course participation, including attendance at sessions outside the institution.

Exhibit 2-8 is an example of reports compiled on educational activities. This is used as the master schedule for courses and to compile specific information about each. The summary sheet (Exhibit 2-9) is prepared at the end of each semester or summer session and totaled annually.

Staff activities in other than planning and implementing courses should be included in departmental reports. These include committee work in organizations; professional memberships and activities; personal development, including nonacademic credit and academic credit work; presentations; publications; awards or grants received; and other information to indicate staff members' accomplishments.

## POLICIES AND PROCEDURES

The continuing education staff operates under the policies and procedures of the overall organization of which it is a part. However, some policies and procedures may need to be altered to meet differences in operation of the education department and others in the organization. Any alterations to meet the operational requirements of the education department should be reviewed and approved by the appropriate administrative bodies. Some policies and procedures may be unique to the department and must be developed specifically for it. They also should be approved by the administration.

All policies and procedures used in the operation of the department should be available to all staff members involved in the program. A manual of policies and procedures is very important to the efficient administration of the program.

### Course Registration and Fees

In a college or university, policies and procedures for registrations for continuing education may be handled the same as they are for all other students. However, there usually are sufficient differences to require the establishment of specific policies and procedures for continuing education in nursing.

**Exhibit 2-8** Compilation Form on Educational Programs

COLUMBUS CAMPUS OF IUPUI
CONTINUING EDUCATION ACTIVITIES

SEMESTER _____ 19 ____    SCHEDULE: DAY/MONTH/DATE    BASIS    RESULTS    SHEET ____ OF ____

| ACTIVITY NUMBER | ACTIVITY TITLE | DAYS-FEE MIN—MAX | CONTACT HOURS | ENROLL MENT | STUDENT CONTACT HOURS | INDIV CEU AWARD | INSTI CEU RECORD | GROSS INCOME |
|---|---|---|---|---|---|---|---|---|
| | | | | | | | | |
| | | | | | | | | |
| | | | | | | | | |
| | | | | | | | | |
| | | | | | | | | |
| | | | | | | | | |
| | | | | | | | | |
| | | | | | | | | |
| | | | | | | | | |
| | | | | | | | | |
| | | | | | | | | |
| | | | | | | | | |
| | | | | | | | | |
| | | | | | | | | |
| | | | | | | | | |
| | | | | | | | | |

TOTALS NURSING

TOTALS GENERAL

TOTAL COMBINED

NOTE:  For explanation of terminology used above see reverse side.

Form adopted 1/80

EXPLANATION OF TERMINOLOGY USED:

1. ENROLLMENT: Total number of individual participants in attendance.

2. CONTACT HOUR: A typical 50 minute classroom instructional session or equivalent.

3. STUDENT CONTACT HOUR: Enrollment times instructor contact hours.

4. CEU: Continuing Education Unit(s) = ten contact hours of participation in an organized Continuing Education experience under responsible sponsorship, capable direction, and qualified instruction.

   INDIVIDUAL CEU: Enrollment times predetermined CEU may be approved for awards to individual participants.

   INSTITUTION CEU: Predetermined CEU not awarded to individuals assigned to the institution.

5. GROSS INCOME: Total dollar income received from Continuing Education activities before any expense deductions.

6. FTE ENROLLMENTS: Full time equivalent = total student contact hours divided by 480 (480 = 15hrs./FTE x 16 wks./semester x 2 sem./yr).

*Source:* Reprinted from *Departmental Operating Manual*, Division of Continuing Studies, Columbus Campus, Indiana University-Purdue University at Indianapolis, © 1980.

**Exhibit 2-9** Example of Activity Summary Sheet

COLUMBUS CAMPUS OF IUPUI

ANNUAL SUMMARY: CONTINUING EDUCATION NURSING ACTIVITIES

| SEMESTER | No. Activities Scheduled | No. Activities Completed | Total Student Contact Hrs. | Total Enrollment | Ind. CEU Awarded | Inst. CEU Recorded | Gross Income | FTE Enrollment | Space for Accumulative If Desired |
|----------|---|---|---|---|---|---|---|---|---|
| SUMMER II | | | | | | | | | |
| FALL | | | | | | | | | |
| SPRING | | | | | | | | | |
| SUMMER I | | | | | | | | | |
| TOTALS FOR YEAR | | | | | | | | | |

*Source:* Reprinted from *Departmental Operating Manual,* Division of Continuing Studies, Columbus Campus, Indiana University-Purdue University at Indianapolis, ©1980.

Policies include methods to be used for fee determination. The program may have an established daily or hourly fee or the figure may be determined individually for each course, based on the cost of the program. **Policies** also need to be established for fee waivers or reductions. For example, persons who assist in the planning of the course or certain individuals such as faculty members in other departments of the school of nursing or nurses in health facilities associated with the school of nursing may be granted waivers or reductions. If there is an additional charge for registration after a certain date, this needs to be stated as a policy. Policies are needed for refunds of registration fees, including the time frame and amount that will be repaid. A percentage of the fee may be retained for the cost incurred in processing the registration and the refund.

Procedures are established to define the process for handling registration, including who is responsible for each step in the process such as recording the registration, depositing the fees to the appropriate account, and issuing receipts. Receipts may be used as acknowledgments to registrants that they are enrolled in the course. Receipts also are useful since continuing education costs are tax deductible.

The policies on registration and fees should be stated in the continuing education brochure or catalog. Registration deadline dates should be stated clearly, particularly if there is an additional fee for late registration.

The staff development department should establish policies and procedures for handling registrations for nurses employed in the institution and for those from other organizations if the courses are open to outside nurses. These will be the same as for the college or university. Since the registration and fee collection processes, unlike those at a college or university, may be unique to the department in a health care facility, the unit's staff will be responsible for writing the policies and procedures and obtaining approvals.

The unit responsible for providing continuing education in nursing in a professional association should develop and recommend policies for registration and fee collection for programs sponsored by the association. Policies should be stated on member and nonmember fees and how these will be determined. Policies on refunds, fee reductions, and late registrations also are needed.

## Payment of Instructors

The process for payment of instructors should comply with the guidelines for payment of other persons employed on a part-time or occasional basis. Guidelines may be established specifically for the amount to be paid faculty members based on their education and experience. Procedures for processing payment or payroll forms may need to be modified to define any areas of differences. For example, the payroll office generally prepares forms for personnel employed in the organization but the forms for faculty in continuing education courses may be the responsibility of the continuing education department. Where multiple forms exist for payment of different classifications of personnel, procedures should indicate how each type is to be used. An example of each form should be included in the policy and procedure manual. For example, if payment is being made to a faculty member from another department in the school, there usually is a specific payroll form that must be used.

## Travel

Travel expenses paid to persons employed in continuing education generally are based on the established policies and procedures of the overall organization. Copies of these rules should be included in the department's policy and procedure manual. The policies should be updated as the institution changes reimbursement rates for mileage, per diem, and other expenses. If mileage is reimbursed on the basis of map figures, it is helpful to include a chart of the distances from different cities in the procedure manual.

## Supplies and Textbooks

Procedures for requisitioning supplies generally are the same for the continuing education department as for all others. The procedure and examples of forms to be used should be in the department's policy and procedure manual. The department may develop additional policies and procedures as deemed necessary. Guidelines for records and reports were discussed previously; others may be established as needed on maintenance of records.

The policies and procedures need to be reviewed and updated periodically. As changes are made in organizational requirements, they should be incorporated in the department manual. All should include the date established and the date of the latest revision.

---

**SUGGESTED READINGS**

Houle, Cyril O. *Continuing Learning in the Professions.* San Francisco: Jossey-Bass, Inc., 1980.

Knox, Alan B., ed. *Enhancing Proficiencies of Continuing Educators.* San Francisco: Jossey-Bass, Inc., Number 1, 1979.

Lauffer, Armand. *Doing Continuing Education and Staff Development.* New York: McGraw-Hill Book Co., 1978.

**Chapter 3**

# Marketing

Marketing of continuing education and staff development activities is a field that is coming into its own. Many educators have felt distinct discomfort in using the terms and procedures of marketing that have long been associated only with commercial enterprises, in part because they have regarded some of the marketing by corporations as bordering on the unethical. Because it may have been misused, however, does not mean that marketing itself does not have redeeming qualities; the difficulty lies in the behavior of those who market rather than in the ethics of the process. Marketing of continuing education will be assumed to take place in an educational environment under the direction of ethical people.

Marketing is an essential component of continuing education sponsorship. Very few education programs have access to public relations experts to assist in marketing their wares. Thus it becomes the responsibility of the program staff to do the marketing. If the staff members are neophytes in marketing knowledge and skill, all too often their efforts emerge as rather amateurish attempts at public relations. It is imperative that the staff become skilled in marketing, since the manner in which the process is approached may well spell the difference between its being a success or a failure.

## MARKETING STRATEGY

The initial step in marketing a continuing education program is to plan a strategy. This marketing strategy is merely setting down and defining the specific elements of a plan.

A marketing strategy should be appropriate to the agency or organization and to its target audience. It is based on the program's philosophy, goals, and objectives. The type of sponsoring organization also affects the strategy.

It is helpful to develop a marketing plan that describes the environment in which the continuing education and staff development courses are conducted. It should include the issues that may impact on the organization's external and internal environment. It should describe policy, directions, and objectives of the total organization and of the continuing education program as well as the means for achieving them. Marketing messages, themes, and media are outlined as well as how much of the department's resources are committed to the strategy, including people, money, and time.

## Identifying the Audience

The strategy assesses the existing market for the program's offerings. To pinpoint this, the potential audience to be served must be identified (and included in the program's mission statement as well). This audience includes:

1. those individuals who are part of the actual market—that is, they currently attend the continuing education events the organization sponsors
2. those individuals who are part of the potential audience—that is, they may attend the courses
3. those individuals who are not interested in or do not need to attend any activities

These audiences will vary from time to time depending upon such factors as the program subject, the time of year, the course location, and so on.

The size of the target audience, its demographic characteristics, the specialty areas represented, and its employment status affect the continuing education program and help determine the parameters of the marketing strategy. The size of the potential audience may be affected by such factors as technology, economics, social changes, skill level requirements, and turnover.

The territory covered by the agency or organization conducting the program also affects the marketing strategy. Examples of territory include (1) a specific catchment area, (2) a local area such as county or district, (3) an urban or rural area, (4) a state, (5) a region, or (6) a national area.

The essential components of a marketing strategy include always being prepared well in advance of the scheduled activity and using the right techniques in preparing promotional materials. The need for accuracy in presenting the program to potential participants goes without saying. Marketing also involves ethical responsibilities. Since much marketing is simply good public relations, politeness and good manners are the watchwords for effectiveness.

## Other Steps in the Process

Marketing goes beyond the procedure of designing and mailing out brochures for a specific activity. The process includes these elements:

- identifying the potential audience, knowing the learners' educational needs, and putting those individuals first in attempting to meet those needs

- planning continuing education activities to meet those identified needs

- publicizing the educational activities to make potential participants aware of their availability

- implementing the activity so that there is an appreciable benefit to the participants

- evaluating the entire process, including the planning, implementing, and promoting, so that future directions can be determined

Once key decisions are made to create a marketing strategy, the next step is to take specific actions to implement it. The entire staff of the continuing education and staff development department should be involved in developing the strategy to ensure its success. The marketing plan is reviewed at least annually, or more often if organizational changes so require, and is revised as often as necessary because an outdated strategy is almost worse than none at all. The plan should include an evaluation of its effectiveness. Staff members may wish to attend a continuing education course on marketing to learn how to develop a plan. Large corporations often develop marketing plans as part of their budgeting process; often these plans are available for review so that they can be used as a model for a continuing education program.

## Four Ps of Marketing

The plan should be based on the elements known as the "Four Ps of Marketing:" (1) Product, (2) Place, (3) Price, and (4) Promotion.

The *product* is the service offered by the continuing education program. Generally that service consists of courses or classes that meet the identified needs of the nurse learners. Beyond that, however, the educational events help nurses to remain current in their practice, enhance their knowledge and skills, and perhaps even help them qualify for promotions or merit raises. The program also often offers counseling services for nurses who wish to continue their education in either an academic or nonacademic setting. In the institution, the staff often provide services such as educational expertise and counseling related to instruction for employees from other departments. This total package of services, as well as others not identified here, is the product of the continuing education department that must be marketed if the program is to be effective.

A broader perspective on the total product will help in defining its market. The target audience often is defined as nurses in certain areas of practice or jobs. In this way, large segments of the nursing population can be overlooked as potential buyers of the program's product. Identification of the product will help market it outside of the institution but the need for promoting it inside the institution should not be overlooked.

The *place* where the continuing education products are available is the second significant element in a marketing plan. More and more educational activities are moving out to where the audience is—for example, courses for academic credit are held in shopping centers. A university can take its courses to a branch or regional campus to make them accessible to nurses in other areas. The continuing education department can take its courses to places where nurses are employed, such as hospitals, nursing homes, and other health care facilities. The program can make increasing use of public facilities, such as motels, hotels, libraries, churches, banks, and shopping centers, to take the product to where the nurses are.

The appropriate place for classes may be determined by the content and teaching methods; for example, if there is a clinical experience component, it would need to be scheduled in a health care facility. Potential learners can be useful in identifying class sites. Other features may enhance a location—child care service for a nurse with children may be attractive. For courses lasting longer than one day, a nearby shopping area, excellent restaurants, and recreational facilities may be an enticement for a nurse to enroll. Family-centered educational activities during the summer in places such as camps or state parks with boating, fishing, and swimming may prove attractive for the prospective audience. For a series of classes, particularly those in the evenings, the place must be selected with a view toward safety as well as parking convenience and eating facilities.

The *price* of an educational offering often is viewed as a deterrent to attendance that could have an impact on marketing. However, in a study of a 10 percent random sample of registered nurses licensed and residing in Indiana on reasons for participation and nonparticipation in continuing education activities, cost was not identified as a major reason for not attending, indicating that perhaps marketing should focus on the quality aspects of the course rather than just its price. Slightly more nurses attended on their own time than entirely on their employers' time. This difference in percentage of personal time spent in continuing education activities was significant at the .001 level. It is unlikely that a difference of this magnitude was due to chance.

Nurses also were asked to indicate the percentage of the total cost of their attendance that was paid by them and/or by their employer. One in every four attenders paid all of the cost of attendance, while one in every three paid none. This difference also was significant at the .001 level.

The respondents also were asked to indicate who paid for specific items of continuing education. The results indicated that the employer tended to pay the registration fee more often than did the nurse, while the nurse paid for transportation, food, and lodging more often than the employer. The nurse also generally paid for materials such as textbooks, stethoscopes, and so on, more often than did the employer.

Many courses or workshops have to generate enough income to cover both direct and indirect costs. Some organizations may be satisfied with recovery of a "reasonable" amount of the cost. Others price the activities to ensure overage, while still others charge only enough to recoup operating costs. The price charged for the course depends in large part on the policies of the institution in which the continuing education department is located. The price can be based on the cost, either indirect or direct, calculated at no more than a break-even point. Sometimes the price may be based on recovery of direct costs only, with indirect expenses such as time and overhead not charged.

Many registration fees purposely are set at minimal levels in the hope of attracting participants, and some even are free. While these prices are based on the notion that nurses are unwilling or unable to pay, this tactic often has the reverse effect. Nurses may not attend because they feel that "it can't be worth anything" if offered free or cheaply.

Overpricing can have the same effect: nurses may attend a course that is highly priced because they think price equals quality. Many times they are mistaken in this assumption and must be educated to select classes that will assist them in meeting their goals rather than relying on price as an index of quality.

The continuing education program can select several approaches to pricing and should vary them depending on the need and potential market. A high fee may be charged the first time a course is offered to recover the planning and implementation costs. When the event is repeated, the fee can be lowered.

Another approach is to base the price on what it is believed the market will bear. If there is a strong need for a course in a particular subject area, then its price may be set a bit higher than for one that does not have as great a demand.

The *promotion* of the services of the continuing education program is the final element of the marketing plan. The recipients of the services, both actual and potential, must be made aware of what is available. Promotional activities can be carried out by the entire program staff or one individual can be assigned the responsibility for all such endeavors.

## Public Relations

One individual in the continuing education program may be designated as the public relations person. That individual can be either a professional staff person or a support staff member interested in public relations. The individual must have several characteristics if implementation of the marketing strategy is to be successful. The public relations person should be involved with the potential audience and should be aware of issues and trends in the professions for which continuing education activities are being provided. Knowledge and skill in communicating with members of the potential audience will enhance the effectiveness of the promotional materials developed.

The public relations person must be realistic and able to accept the internal or external limitations on the continuing education program. It is not effective to plan to spend money in excess of what has been budgeted for promotion. The individual chosen must be given control over the public relations effort. If there are decisions to be made, that person—and only that person— should make them.

### Creativity an Essential

The public relations person should be creative, imaginative, and maybe a bit daring in implementing the marketing strategy; innovative approaches can increase the size of the audience. The person should be daring enough to try nontraditional ways of publicizing the program as long as they remain within the bounds of good taste.

The public relations individual should be prepared to implement the marketing strategy for a particular course well in advance of its being offered. Deadlines must be established and adhered to. Preparation allows others to count on receiving promotional materials at the appropriate time so that there will be no delays on the part of the printer, the mail room, or others involved in the marketing plan. The public relations person must be organized and accurate in work habits. Last-minute crises can occur but should not be a way of life. Brochures should not be sent out with missing information, and so on. The individual should establish and maintain checklists for promotional activities to decrease the possibility of missing deadlines or making errors.

Finally, the person must keep good records so that when the individual is absent, questions and problems involving the marketing plan can be handled by others in the continuing education program. The other staff members also should be able to tell at a glance where the marketing plan for a particular course stands at a given time. For example, if a nurse calls to ask when a particular class will be scheduled, any staff member should be able to give the date and indicate that "brochures will be sent out in two weeks—they are now at the printer."

## *Involvement in Planning*

The public relations person should be involved in the planning process for each course sponsored by the program so as to be aware of the focus of the event, the target audience, and what is likely to attract potential participants. Because it may be difficult to attend planning meetings for many offerings, the person may wish to form a task force of volunteers to provide assistance in the public relations effort.

In addition to serving on the various planning committees, members of the task force for public relations may offer advice and assistance on promotional methods for specific events. The task force can be composed of experts in various public relations areas so that the program individual can obtain much of value from their knowledge. Individuals who work with chambers of commerce, voluntary health organizations, or other similar entities often are willing to assist the public relations efforts of a continuing education staff. A person in the public relations business may serve on a task force. If the program is university based, the expert may serve because of being an alumnus; if it is hospital based, the person may serve because of having been a patient.

Having a member of the public relations task force or the public relations person in the department on each planning committee will help keep publicity proposals more realistic. Planning committees should be made aware of the costs of publicity. The expense may be calculated not only in terms of the paper, printing, and postage but also in terms of the cost of the time required by the public relations person and support staff to promote a particular offering successfully. This becomes an especially critical consideration since the public relations person may not be doing such work full-time and have other duties, so that this function is sandwiched into a busy schedule. The public relations person thus must be highly organized and make efficient use of available time. The planning committee and those utilizing the services of the public relations person also must be aware of the time constraints. Involving someone from the task force early in the planning stage will allow the public relations person to set priorities and prepare effective publicity.

## MARKETING TECHNIQUES

Many marketing techniques are available. Some will prove more successful than others; experience based on trial and error generally is the best way of determining what works in a given situation.

## Advertising

General marketing techniques include advertisements: continuing education events can be advertised in journals, calendars, and newspapers. Some professional journals will list upcoming continuing education activities free but others may impose a small charge. A first step is to write the journals of choice for their policies on advertising of continuing education events. Advertising should be placed in the journal most likely to be read by the target audience. For courses aimed at the general nursing population, the journals with the largest readership should be used. Journals have specific deadline dates for submission of advertising copy. These deadlines are absolute and must be adhered to.

When preparing copy for a specific journal, it is a good idea to obtain several back issues to study the style of the advertisements it carries. If the advertisement is patterned after those already published, the copy writer may well save doing some work. At the minimum, advertisements should consist of the title of the educational activity, the sponsoring organization, the location, date, time, regulations for registration (including deadline for preregistration, whether there is onsite registration), fees and what they cover, who the target audience is, who the speakers are, and any other features that make this event attractive.

Calendars of continuing education events are published by many sponsors of such activities. State nurses' associations often issue calendars particularly for their membership. It may be possible to advertise free, or for a small fee, in such calendars or in other material sent to the associations' membership.

Organizations such as the chamber of commerce or convention bureau often publish lists of activities in a city and can include continuing education activities, particularly those of interest to a large segment of the nursing population.

Several multistate calendars of continuing education events are published by commercial firms. Paid advertisements can be placed in these publications, particularly if the activity is likely to appeal to nurses in several states.

Newspaper advertisements also can be used as a marketing technique. If another department in the organization also is advertising in the local newspaper, it may be possible to "piggyback" with that department and substantially reduce costs. Newspapers often offer a reduced nonprofit or educational institution advertising rate; it is worthwhile to inquire about the cost.

When considering newspaper advertising, it is wise to investigate using the small suburban weeklies near most major cities. Advertising in such newspapers costs considerably less than in metropolitan dailies. The small newspapers may reach a particular audience more effectively; for example, when a return-to-nursing refresher course is planned, the nurse-housewife may be reached more effectively with a suburban newspaper than with the metro daily.

## Broadcasting

Publicity through the broadcast media can take the form of paid advertising or free coverage. Paid advertising has been described for newspapers but it also is available on television or radio. Broadcast commercials can be expensive, depending upon the time at which they are to be aired. Commercials that continuing education budgets can afford seldom are broadcast at times that will ensure the desired audience. Rates vary for both radio and television, so they should be investigated carefully before ads are placed.

Free coverage is available on both radio and television if what is being publicized is news. If a continuing education event is something that is of interest to many persons, it can be considered news. The education information should be something that will affect the people in the community, such as when nurses are learning how to be effective in natural disasters (floods, tornadoes, etc.). A topic involving local residents also is considered news, such as when a nurse from a community is to be a faculty leader for an educational course. Newspapers and radio stations in small towns are well known for publishing such information of local interest.

News is something unusual that is happening in the community. Bringing in a "name" speaker is an event that the media consider news. Educational offerings that focus on community events may be considered news, such as when an important football game is held in the city, and concurrently there is an educational session on "Nursing Management of Sports Injuries."

## Use of the News Release

Information provided to the media about continuing education activities should consist of the what, who, where, why, when, and how. Other specifics can be added to the news release that is written and distributed to area media sources (Exhibit 3-1). A news release should be brief but contain all of the essential information about the educational program, including who to contact for more information. The release should be written in such a way that it can be used as is by the media; they should not have to rewrite—releases that need to be rewritten completely tend to end up in the wastebasket.

These same releases can be provided to the participants at an educational event who then can insert their names and submit the release to their local newspapers. As mentioned previously, newspapers in small towns often publish information of local interest that larger newspapers would overlook. Participants should be asked to send in copies of any newspaper articles; this will help refine target sources for future releases.

**Exhibit 3-1** Example of a News Release

FROM:
News Bureau
Indiana University Northwest
3400 Broadway
Gary, IN 46408
AC 219, 980-6800
June 10, 1980

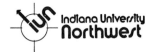
Indiana University
Northwest

FOR IMMEDIATE RELEASE                                    WORKSHOP ON LEGAL
                                                        ASPECTS OF NURSING

Legal aspects of contemporary nursing practice will be the subject of a one-day workshop June 25 for both registered and licensed practical nurses.  The 8:30 a.m. - 4 :30 p.m. session will be held in the Harvest Room at Southlake Mall as part of the Indiana University Northwest Continuing Nursing Education Program.

Mary D. Hemelt, who is both a nurse and a lawyer and who is acting associate dean and professor of allied health at Essex Community College in Baltimore, will teach the course.  She is also co-author of Dynamics of Law in Nursing and Health Care.

The workshop, for which participants can earn 0.7 continuing education units, will cover medical negligence liability in relation to nursing responsibility for a dignified death, resuscitation and organ harvesting.  It will also examine legal responsibilities in nursing administration and such current concerns in nursing practice as rape, abortion, child abuse, splitting medications, and misdiagnosis.

Legal and ethical implications of the nurse's responsibilities for patients' rights, plus advocacy, counselling, and student, staff, and patient education will also be reviewed.

Complete registration information is available from the continuing nursing education office at IUN   Phone: 980-6604 or 980-6605.

-TJB-

*Source:* Reprinted by permission of Indiana University Northwest, Gary, Indiana, 1980.

When sending out a press release, it is most effective to direct it to an individual by name. Identifying the appropriate individual should be the first step in determining which media sources are likely targets for publicity efforts.

A well-written, eye-catching news release may result in an inquiry for further information from the media. Radio and television talk shows interview individuals who are making news. In such an interview, the continuing education efforts can be discussed. Again, many of these programs may be on the air in other than prime time but still may attract potential learners. Newspapers may do a feature article on the educational event. Many newspapers list coming events such as continuing education activities on a space-available basis.

The media often carry information on educational programs as public service announcements. These should be brief but contain enough information that potential learners can decide whether the event is appropriate for them and also find out who to contact for more details. These public service announcements (PSAs) often are broadcast at off times and so may not be all that effective for drawing large numbers, but every bit of publicity helps.

In every instance, the material submitted for a public service announcement or listing should be brief and to the point. PSAs should not be longer than half a minute or about 50 words. The writer must be certain to include the what, who, when, where, why, and how, as well as the name, address, and telephone number of the person to be contacted for more information. Information for a public service announcement or listing should be sent to the media at least two to three weeks before it is to be used.

In all these materials, the language used is important. The writer must avoid any language that could be in poor taste (such as sexist), that has double meanings, or that is jargon known only by those in the trade.

## DIRECT MAIL TECHNIQUES

Direct mail techniques can be the most successful component of a marketing strategy. Direct mail is a popular method that is easy to implement, attractive, and can be fairly easily maintained as part of the continuing education program to hold down time and money costs. To be effective, however, direct mail must be well designed and reach the audience for which it is intended.

## Mailing Lists

For the direct mail pieces to reach the largest segment of the target population, the education program must develop and maintain an up-to-date and complete mailing list. The list can be designed to include individual nurses and agencies and organizations that employ or represent them. Establishing a mailing list is a time-consuming and costly project but must be accomplished as part of the marketing strategy. Once established, it can be relatively easy to maintain.

A beginning for a mailing list for nurses in a state or a particular geographic area is the state board of nurses' registration. Restrictions on releasing the names and addresses of licensed nurses vary in each state so contact must be made with the board well in advance of the time the mailing list is needed. Professional organizations for nurses at national, state, or local levels have membership lists that they may (or may not) make available. Often there is a charge for such lists to cover the cost of the labels on which the names are printed. If an educational event is being cosponsored with another organization, the latter may share its mailing list. Voluntary health organizations have mailing lists of their members. For example, mental health associations and the Red Cross may be willing to share their lists, either free or for a fee.

It is essential that the marketing planners be honest about what they intend to do with the mailing lists. If the lists are to be used for a one-time mailing for a specific course or workshop, it is not ethical to incorporate all of those names into the program's master mailing list. The lists from organizations and agencies that charge for them should be purchased each time a mailing to that target group is planned; those names should not be used for any purpose beyond the one identified when the list was requested.

The mailing list should be tested to determine its accuracy. One mailing should be done first class, so that returns will indicate change of address, moved, and so on. The list then should be corrected.

Maintaining a mailing list requires continuous attention. It should be updated at least twice a year. Additions can be made from rosters of participants and from their inquiries. These persons also can be asked to supply the names of others who might be interested in order to expand the list. Once a list is compiled and tested, mailings can be made at rates less expensive than first class. Rising postage costs make mailing at bulk rate more attractive, although the cost benefit may be offset by the slower delivery rate.

Two major types of direct mail pieces are the catalog and the single item.

## Catalogs

A catalog requires long-term advance planning of educational events (perhaps a year) if it is to be a cost-effective means of advertising. The catalog is the best means of advertising broad general listings of forthcoming programs. It is best directed toward a broad general audience, such as all of the nurses in a geographic area. A catalog can help individuals who are accustomed to attending some form of educational course or workshop to plan ahead.

A major value of a catalog is that it is retained by the receiver, who may go through it several times. A single piece may be scanned only briefly, then discarded if not thought appropriate. It also is limited in scope in comparison to a catalog. Some combination of catalog listings followed by a single-piece mailing probably is best in most instances.

## Single-Piece Mailing

A single piece is best for a new offering, for one focused on a specific topic, or for an easily identified audience, such as members of a specialty nursing organization or in a particular area of clinical practice. A single piece also is useful in responding to inquiries generated by a catalog. More recent and more specific information can be contained in a single piece than may have been available when a catalog was prepared—such as room locations, cost of required texts, and other details. Single-piece mailings also are called offering brochures.

## Persuasive Communication in Mailings

Direct mailings for a specific educational offering are a form of persuasive communication. The object is to persuade the recipient to attend that particular course. There are many ways to develop persuasive communication skills. A simple formula is A I D A: attention, interest, desire, action. Keeping this formula in mind as brochures are being designed will help the marketing effort become more successful.

### Attention

It is essential to get the recipient's attention immediately before the person decides to throw the brochure away. Something about the brochure should capture attention, whether it is the color, the printing, the type, the design, the title of the workshop, or something else. The headline or lead should be related to the recipient's needs or interests. The title is extremely important in attracting attention: "How to," "Announcing," "Learn to," and "Advice."

### Interest

Once the recipient's attention is on the brochure, the next step is to maintain interest. The message should be expanded by pointing out the benefit of attending the course. This can be accomplished by highlighting the workshop objectives, which are written in terms of what the participant will (or should) be able to do at the completion of the event.

*Desire*

The next step is to persuade the recipient that what the brochure promises actually will occur. This can be accomplished by including the program outline to demonstrate how the content and methods will help in the achievement of the objectives.

*Action*

This is the point at which the recipient reaches a decision about attending the activity. The recipient should be told exactly what to do: "Complete the registration form TODAY." The means for taking that action, such as a tear-off registration form, should be provided. The best registration form is one that can be removed from the brochure without having to tear off valuable information such as objectives, content, method, faculty, date, time, and place.

Another useful formula in persuasive communication is used by a large and very successful consumer advertising agency. The formula consists of four steps:

1. **Know the prime prospects.** Know who is a possible attender at the educational offerings; know what the audience is like and how it differs from those of other sponsors of such activities. These data can be collected by a thorough review of the demographic data collected on past participants or by developing a new survey to assess the target audience.

2. **Know the prime prospects' problems.** What are they concerned about and what might they be interested in learning about? A needs survey will provide this information.

3. **Know the product or service being offered.** What does the program have to offer prime prospects, who else offers the same service, how do they differ?

4. **Break the boredom barrier.** Communicate to the audience in a manner that is different from how competitors do so. How can this program communicate what it has to offer in a way that sets it apart from all of the other communications received by the potential audience?

One way to provide that difference is to stress the benefits the participants will receive from this program. This responds to the "What's in it for me?" question. People do not buy a product, service, or idea—they buy the benefits of that product, service, or idea. If the brochures indicate the benefits to be gained by attendance, the participants won't have to determine that themselves or, even worse, misinterpret the benefits and, after attending, feel they have been "ripped off" because the implied results were not delivered.

## Benefit Profile

Focusing on the uniqueness of the offerings is part of an effective marketing strategy that can identify the benefits of a particular educational event. It also is essential to identify sponsors of other similar workshops or courses and determine how this program is unique in comparison to theirs.

The individuals who helped plan the program may provide a somewhat biased view of what is unique, so if possible individuals who do not have any experience with the event should be included. They should be given as much information as possible about the program, then encouraged to come up with fresh, new ideas using a brainstorming approach. When all of the ideas of uniqueness are recorded, the leader asks "So what?" about each idea. When all of the "so whats" are answered, the benefit to the potential attender should be clear. For example, if the course is sponsored by a hospital for employees only, the unique idea is that it will carry approved continuing education units (CEU). "So what?" may lead to the conclusion that nurses can earn those CEU in their employment setting, which should be a convenience. So what? It will minimize the time lost for transportation and will reduce the cost since the nurses won't have to pay for hotel rooms and meeting space. When there are no unanswered "so whats?" then a benefit has been pinpointed. The benefit identified can be made an important part of communication with the potential audience. For example, "You can avoid all the hassle of driving to a continuing education offering and earn CEU as you learn," can be the lead in the brochure.

This exercise can bring out other unique aspects of the program. The next step is to combine the benefits identified in the communication with the potential audience. Elements to look for include benefits related to content, faculty, methods, and other factors. The benefit list changes with every event, so each should be profiled separately. If persons who have not participated in the planning are involved in the benefit profile process, their inclusion serves the additional purpose of generating enthusiasm about the program that they then can communicate to others.

## Brochure Design

The easiest kind of brochure to design and distribute is a standard three-fold that can be mailed without having to be inserted into an envelope. On the reverse side of the fold bearing the address label is the registration form, which registrants return. Both sides of the two other folds contain information about the what, who, where, when, why, and how of the workshop or course.

The design of the single-piece mailing is important. People are conscious about design more than ever because they are stimulated by new styles in almost everything almost daily. Design conveys to the participants how the sponsors conceive of the offering; the design reflects the institution (or program) and the value it places on the course. Brochures that receive little attention are those crammed with information typed or, even worse, handwritten (and not too legibly). Expert typesetting gives a professional look, but a superslick brochure may be overkill.

A professional graphic designer can be used to develop a basic format for the continuing education program; that format is followed for each brochure. The design can be preprinted on several colors of paper, rotated for each new event, on which copy can be presented describing a specific activity. Such format standardization makes it easier to prepare brochures each time a workshop is planned, but a problem occurs when the mailings become indistinguishable to the recipient, one from another.

The color of the brochure should be different each time so that the recipient doesn't think it is a duplicate of an earlier one. The key here is to use a wide variety of colors of paper, not just three or four. Paper is available in colors that vary from the standard blues and greens to fuschia and orchid.

It also is worthwhile to consider varying the color of ink. This can add somewhat to the cost of the printing, however, so it should be evaluated as to whether the benefit justifies the additional expense.

An inexpensive variation is in the size and style of type. This can be done by a professional typesetter or by using interchangeable typefaces on an office typewriter. Again caution is necessary so that these variations are not overdone, which may detract from rather than enhance the appearance of the brochure.

The design of the brochure can be carried over to the cover of the catalog, the folders for participants' handouts, letterheads, and so on. This carry-over of the design will ensure instant identification of the continuing education program.

The brochure should be designed to contain a registration form that is simple to complete. It should not ask for more information than absolutely necessary to process the registration. If part of the mission of the program is research in continuing education, then it may be desirable to collect demographic data on participants. That task is best accomplished on the day of the workshop or course when this intent can be announced and participants' cooperation solicited. Participants who are requested to include their nursing license or registration number, educational background, and so on may find completing the registration form a chore, and so may not complete it just because of its complexity. A registration process should be as easy as possible for the nurse. Registration by phone or payment of fees by credit card may increase the number of nurses who enroll.

Advertisements for the event should include premiums that the enrollee will get for attending. If the fee covers a textbook, for example, that should be identified clearly. A caution here is that what is promised must be delivered; if each participant is to receive a copy of the textbook "absolutely free" and the copies do not arrive from the publisher in time, the program will lose credibility with that audience.

Whether the brochure is printed professionally or prepared in-house, it cannot be proofread enough. It is disastrous for a brochure to be mailed lacking some of the essential information about a course. Because the planners, program staff, and public relations person are so familiar with the activity, they may easily overlook vital information the participant needs in order to decide whether to attend.

Several fairly common mistakes in brochures occur when particulars about registration are omitted, such as deadlines or time of day; sometimes, the day of the week and the date do not coincide. Fairly common also is the misspelling of the names of faculty or planning committee members.

## Mailing

Timing for mailings is important. Most organizations mail in September, December, and April, the fewest in August, July, and October. The continuing education program should decide whether to mail with the crowd or in the off months. If the event has limited appeal to a rather small audience, then competition is not a problem and the mailing date is not an issue in this respect. If the program is on a currently popular topic that will result in competition, then it is better to mail when others aren't. The general mailing trends in the area can be determined by analyzing the flow of educational flyers across the desk. When do most of them come? What are the heaviest mailing months? What are the lightest?

Analysis of others' educational brochures will produce numerous design ideas. However, it is essential not to copy too closely, or the program's flyers will resemble those of the competition.

A preannouncement may be advisable if the brochure is being mailed when many others are. The preannouncement can spark interest by indicating there is a workshop coming that's worth waiting for, and recipients will watch for the brochures. The brochure mailing can be varied by sending a letter of no more than two pages, with the registration blank at the bottom of the second page. This format will be successful if the copy is informative, crisp, and does not oversell the event. The format can be varied.

Another form of premailing is a postcard that describes a specific program or serves as a reminder after the regular brochure has been sent. Postcards offer variety in mailing and can be designed in a style similar to the brochures to provide recognition.

Peak days at the post office are Friday and Monday, with Tuesday the slowest, so mailings should be planned accordingly.

Mailings should be sent out about eight weeks before the educational event to allow time for agency clearance, participants' requests for time off, and processing registrations. Because many brochures are circulated with the label panel up (rather than the front cover), pertinent information should be repeated on the back to be sure it is noticed. If the back panel doesn't have room for much information, at least the title and perhaps the faculty for the workshop should be listed.

## OTHER PROMOTIONAL METHODS

The continuing education program should take advantage of all opportunities to publicize its workshops, courses, etc.

### Word of Mouth

Word of mouth may be the most effective means of attracting participants. Persons in the target profession should be included on advisory or planning committees. This provides the advantage of having an opinion leader helping with publicity. Advisory and planning committee members are excellent word-of-mouth advocates for continuing education activities in which they have been involved.

### Personal Contact

In all activities in which staff members are involved, they are representing the program. The image of the program that they reflect can be a persuasive marketing technique. In any role, such as consultant, teacher, or facilitator, staff members can market the services of the program. Using contacts made through daily activities, staff members can increase attendance at the workshops or courses. Personal contacts and telephone calls can increase attendance to the point where cancellation for lack of enrollment can be averted.

### Brochure Distribution

Making the brochures available to sources other than those on the mailing list can increase the audience. Members of the advisory and planning committees should be encouraged to distribute the brochures to individuals with whom they come in contact. Brochures can be posted on bulletin boards in agencies or organizations that employ members of the target audience or in supermarkets, drugstores, discount stores, and other places where target learners can see them. Staff members should be encouraged to distribute brochures at meetings they attend, either as participants or as guest speakers.

Exhibits can be used at conventions or other large meetings of target groups. There are conventions of nurses' associations and specialty nursing organizations at state and national levels. Libraries, both public and those associated with colleges or universities, often will permit displays of educational brochures. Voluntary health agencies, American Red Cross chapters, and so on may permit displays of educational brochures, particularly if the topic is related to their focus.

## Records

When promotional materials about educational offerings are distributed, records should be kept to include sources to whom publicity was directed. A checklist for this purpose can be designed to include the number of copies of the brochure printed, addresses, and the cost of the printing and mailing. Other means of brochure distribution also should be recorded, such as the number of copies given to advisory and planning committee members, numbers distributed at which meetings, and the number posted on bulletin boards and where. Publicity related to press releases and their recipients should be listed.

## Publicity Mix

This recordkeeping system can illustrate the mix of publicity means used for educational events. The best mix can be determined by asking participants how they learned of the workshop or course they are attending.

This question should be part of every evaluation form completed by participants. The responses will help determine the most effective marketing techniques for that particular activity. The question may call for a forced-choice response, such as a list of possible sources such as catalog, brochure, word of mouth, journal advertisement, public service announcement, and others. The question can be open ended: how or where the respondent learned of the event, without the staff's suggesting possible sources from which the participant selects.

Matching the program with the manner in which the participants hear of it will provide focus for publicity for future similar events. For example, if the majority of those in attendance learned of the event from a professional journal and the program was targeted toward nurses in a specialty area, a mass mailing of brochures for this kind of workshop may be less effective than a few well-placed advertisements. If nurses heard of a refresher course over the radio, the value of newspaper coverage can be minimized when such events are offered again. In this way, the best advertising sources can be determined and efforts concentrated on them. At the same time, it is important to continue to explore other opportunities to publicize the activities.

## Telephone Inquiries

Most advertising methods will spark inquiries. Each telephone inquiry should be handled courteously and efficiently. The individual responsible for answering the telephone should be knowledgeable about upcoming continuing education activities so that callers may receive the most up-to-date information.

The person answering the telephone should keep a log of inquiries. The log should include the nature of the inquiry, the name and address of the caller so that the individual can be added to the mailing list, and where the person learned of the course. In this way, individual contacts can be made for advertising future educational events.

## Final Task

A final task for the program staff is to thank those involved in the publicity for the workshop or course. These thank-yous are essential to promote good will and increase public relations efforts on the program's behalf in the future. Radio, television, and newspapers that publicized the offering in whatever manner can be thanked briefly but sincerely, which keeps the lines of communication open for the next time publicity will be sought. Members of the task force who helped with the public relations effort should be thanked in writing.

All of the persons involved in whatever way in the marketing should know that their efforts were appreciated. Such courtesies help ensure that they will be willing to expend similar time and energy on future educational events.

## NOTES

Belinda E. Puetz, "Differences Between Indiana Registered Nurse Attenders and Non-Attenders in Continuing Education in Nursing Activities." Mimeographed. (Bloomington, Ind.: Indiana University, 1978).

American Nurses' Association, *Manual of Accreditation of Continuing Education in Nursing* (Kansas City, Mo., 1980), p. 63.

## SUGGESTED READINGS

Boyd, Harper W., Jr., and Massey, William F. *Marketing Management*. New York: Harcourt-Brace-Jovanovich, 1972.

Kotler, Philip. *Marketing for Nonprofit Organizations*. Englewood Cliffs, N.J.: Prentice-Hall, Inc., 1975.

# Chapter 4

# Assessing Needs and Planning Learning Activities

Based on the description of adult learners (in Chapter 1) as individuals who enter class with an orientation toward acquiring solutions to their problems, it is easy to see that programming based on identified needs will facilitate their entrance into the educational situation. The continuing education and staff development program planner must guard against the tendency to provide solutions to "obvious" problems without taking the time necessary to define what they are. Too often the tendency is to provide the answer to apparent learning needs without finding the appropriate question. A careful assessment of the learning needs of the target audience can provide direction to the educational program planner that would be sorely lacking otherwise.

## LEARNING NEEDS OF THE ADULT

Learning needs can be defined as basic wants or desires. Learner needs are differentiated from learner interests, which are likings or preferences. Needs are a requirement while interests are more peripheral to the individual's basic inclinations. Needs and interests are correlated closely and often operate simultaneously in the individual.

When a need is perceived by an adult learner, it can be described as a "felt" need. If someone else identifies a need for an adult learner, it can be called an "ascribed" need. Either one can be a real need. On the other hand, if the situation would not be improved by meeting the need, then, whether felt or ascribed, it is not a real need. Often felt needs are considered symptoms of a problem rather than the real problem. Felt needs can be synonymous with real needs, but not always.

A common tendency of program planners, particularly beginners, is to assume that they know what adults need to learn. While many times that may be correct, all too often the planners are not completely accurate in this assumption and the recommended offering fails for lack of participation. It is better to take the time to assess a target audience's need for the content proposed than to cancel a workshop because not enough people attend to make it financially feasible. All program planning based on identified learner needs is not guaranteed success, but tends to be more attractive than material not based on such needs.

Those assessing needs must take into consideration their constantly changing nature. Needs are not fixed, so their assessment must be a continuing concern.

## METHODS OF ASSESSING LEARNER NEEDS

There are many methods of assessing learner needs. Some continuing education planners may choose a single method to the exclusion of others; others may select a variety of ways. The choice depends on the planner's personal preference as well as on the audience whose needs are being assessed. Other considerations include the financial and people resources available to do the needs assessment.

If a variety of data gathering techniques, such as questionnaires, observations, and interviews, reveal similar learning needs, then the validity of those sources is verified, as is the existence of a real need.

A formal needs assessment should be conducted at the origination of a program and at specified intervals thereafter. An annual comprehensive needs assessment can provide direction for programming for the entire year, with the target audience's needs evaluated as appropriate throughout the ensuing year. For example, if the target audience is registered nurses living in a metropolitan area, a needs assessment of that group would be undertaken at the beginning of the program's fiscal year. During the year, neurosurgical nurses might request that a course be conducted for them. To determine what would be the most appropriate content for that group, a specific assessment of the learning needs of neurosurgical nurses would take place.

### Questionnaire/Survey

A questionnaire is perhaps the most common method for gathering data on needs. Survey tools can be designed in several ways: a forced-choice questionnaire allows the adult to select one of several categories of content needs; an open-ended questionnaire provides more latitude in response but can be more difficult to collate. An example of the latter is a survey form designed in a sentence completion manner, such as, "If I could learn more about my job, I would like most to learn . . . ."

A combination of the two types can be used, with the respondent asked to select a topic from a general content area, then to indicate specifically what material would be useful within that larger area. For example, under the content area need "oncology nursing," the respondent would indicate "chemotherapy" or "dealing with the grief of families." Surveys can be constructed to assess needs over the entire body of knowledge required for the practice of the profession (Exhibit 4-1). Needs surveys also can be constructed that are specific to a particular area of that practice (Exhibit 4-2).

Survey forms can be designed by an individual or by a group. A group obviously will provide more input. Some group members also may assist in the distribution of the survey and compilation of its results.

It is advisable to conduct a pilot test of the survey to ensure completeness and clarity. It is frustrating to design and distribute a survey only to find, when the returns are in, that the data are all but useless. A pilot test on 10 to 12 potential recipients of the survey is adequate. Each individual should complete the form and also answer such questions as, "How long did it take to complete?" "Which questions were unclear?" "How would you improve the questionnaire?" "Were any subject areas missing? If so, what?" When the results of the pilot study are in, changes can be made to improve the form.

It is helpful to ask a group to review the results of the pilot test, since the designer of the survey may have a bias toward it and may not be aware that changes are necessary. This problem virtually is eliminated if a group has been involved in the design. If the changes are rather comprehensive, there should be a second pilot test. In that event, some of the initial group of respondents should reply, in addition to nurses who were not in the original survey.

Although time consuming, this pilot method will help ensure that the ultimate data are valid and useful for program planning.

A well-designed survey instrument can be used for many years. There is no need to design one for each annual needs assessment; minor amendments can be made as changes occur in the knowledge needed by the target population.

The advantages of the questionnaire include ease in data collection and availability of written data to substantiate the assessed needs. Surveys also reach larger groups than can many other methods. The data can be summarized and reported easily. The disadvantages of this method include the cost of the data collection and analysis. A mail questionnaire may yield a low return rate, and care must be taken to select a sample of individuals who are representative of the target population.

**Exhibit 4-1** Example of Broad-Scale Questionnaire: Council on Continuing Education Needs Survey

PLEASE DO NOT PUT YOUR NAME ON THIS SURVEY

A. ☐☐☐☐☐ Please print your zip code in box to left:

Questions B through L are multiple choice with the choices numbered. Please write the number of the answer that applies to you on the line to the left of the question. For example, on question B, if you are a diploma graduate, you'd write: #1. Write only one (1) number on each line.

B. ___ Basic (Initial) Educational Preparation in Nursing:

1. Diploma in Nursing
2. Associate Degree in Nursing
3. Baccalaureate Degree in Nursing

C. ___ Highest Level of Education Completed:

1. Diploma in Nursing
2. Associate Degree in Nursing
3. Associate Degree in Other Field
4. Baccalaureate in Nursing
5. Baccalaureate in Other Field
6. Master's in Nursing
7. Master's in Other Field
8. Doctorate in Nursing
9. Doctorate in Other Field

D. ___ Identify the type of work setting in which you are employed.

1. Community Health Agency
2. Skilled Nursing Facility
3. Hospital
4. Industry
5. Voluntary Health Agency
6. Office
7. Private Practice
8. School Health Service
9. School of Nursing
10. Psychiatric Facility
11. Unemployed or Inactive
12. Other: Please Specify _____

E. ___ What is your area of clinical practice?

1. Community Health
2. Emergency Care
3. Geriatrics
4. Maternity
5. Medical Surgical
6. Mental Health
7. Pediatrics
8. Operating Room
9. Education & Training
10. I.C.U./C.C.U.
11. Rehabilitation
12. No specific clinical area
13. Other: Please Specify _____

F. ___ What type of position do you hold?

1. Administrator or Assistant
2. Consultant
3. Supervisor
4. Head Nurse or Assistant
5. Instructor in School of Nursing
6. Staff Nurse
7. Nursing Education Administrator
8. Inservice Educator
9. Clinical Specialist
10. Discharge Planning Nurse
11. Charge Nurse

12. Researcher
13. Nurse Practitioner
14. Retired Nurse
15. Not Employed
16. Other: Please specify _____

G. ___ How many continuing education in nursing courses, workshops, etc., have you participated in during the last two years?

1. None
2. One or two
3. Three to four
4. Five or more

H. ___ If home study materials and/or learning modules were available, would you be interested in using them?

1. Strongly interested
2. Interested
3. Not very interested
4. Not interested at all

I. ___ What are your usual working hours?

1. Days
2. Evenings
3. Nights
4. Rotate

J. ___ What type of continuing education offering would you most prefer to attend?

1. One day workshop
2. Series of one day workshops over several months
3. Two day workshop
4. Weeklong workshop
5. Evening series weekly over several weeks
6. Interrupted series
7. Other: Please Specify _____
_____

K. ___ What is the best time for you to attend continuing education offerings?

1. Mornings
2. Afternoons
3. Evenings
4. Weekends

L. ___ What is the best day for you to attend continuing education offerings?

1. Monday
2. Tuesday
3. Wednesday
4. Thursday
5. Friday
6. Saturday

M. Currently, if you are interested in obtaining information about continuing education in nursing, what are your main sources of information (Check all which apply to you)

___ Direct mailings from organizations providing courses
___ Other nurses
___ Information provided by employing organizations
___ Local educational institution catalogues and flyers
___ Professional journals and newsletters
___ Other: Please Specify _____

N. The following is a list of possible subject areas for continuing education programming. Please check ONLY those you would seriously consider attending on the line representing the level of content you desire (this is not meant to be exhaustive)

LEVEL OF SUBJECT CONTENT

| | | | |
|---|---|---|---|
| Basic | Intermediate | Advanced | **CLINICAL NURSING** |
| ___ | ___ | ___ | Respiratory · Medical |
| ___ | ___ | ___ | Respiratory · Surgical |
| ___ | ___ | ___ | Cardiovascular · Medical |
| ___ | ___ | ___ | Cardiovascular · Surgical |
| ___ | ___ | ___ | Congenital Heart Disorders |
| ___ | ___ | ___ | Hematologic |
| ___ | ___ | ___ | Mouth, Neck, Esophagus · Medical |
| ___ | ___ | ___ | Mouth, Neck, Esophagus · Surgical |
| ___ | ___ | ___ | Gastric · Medical |
| ___ | ___ | ___ | Gastric · Surgical |
| ___ | ___ | ___ | Intestinal · Medical |
| ___ | ___ | ___ | Intestinal · Surgical |
| ___ | ___ | ___ | Liver and Biliary Tract · Medical |
| ___ | ___ | ___ | Liver and Biliary Tract · Surgical |
| ___ | ___ | ___ | Renal Problems |
| ___ | ___ | ___ | Dialysis |
| ___ | ___ | ___ | Reproductive System · Medical |
| ___ | ___ | ___ | Reproductive System · Surgical |
| ___ | ___ | ___ | Breasts · Medical |
| ___ | ___ | ___ | Breasts · Surgical |
| ___ | ___ | | Dermatologic Problems |
| ___ | ___ | | Burns |
| ___ | ___ | | Plastic Reconstructive Surgery |
| ___ | ___ | | Allergy |
| ___ | ___ | | Endocrine Disorders · Medical |
| ___ | ___ | | Endocrine Disorders · Surgical |
| ___ | ___ | | Eye · Medical |
| ___ | ___ | | Eye · Surgical |
| ___ | ___ | | Ear and Mastoid · Medical |
| ___ | ___ | | Ear and Mastoid · Surgical |
| ___ | ___ | | Nervous System · Medical |
| ___ | ___ | | Nervous System · Surgical |
| ___ | ___ | | Musculoskeletal System · Medical |
| ___ | ___ | | Musculoskeletal System · Surgical |
| ___ | ___ | | Communicable Disease · Pediatric |
| ___ | ___ | | Communicable Disease · Adult |
| ___ | ___ | | Emergency and Disaster Conditions |
| ___ | ___ | | Oncology (specify) _____ |
| ___ | ___ | | Family Planning |
| ___ | ___ | | Genetic Counseling |
| ___ | ___ | | Normal Pregnancy and Delivery |
| ___ | ___ | | High Risk Pregnancy |
| ___ | ___ | | Complications of Pregnancy and Delivery |
| ___ | ___ | | Normal Newborn |
| ___ | ___ | | High Risk Newborn |
| ___ | ___ | | Pediatric Nursing · Medical |
| ___ | ___ | | Pediatric Nursing · Surgical |
| ___ | ___ | | Geriatric Nursing (specify) ___ ___ |
| ___ | ___ | | Community Health Nursing (specify) _____ |
| ___ | ___ | | Psych Mental Health Nursing (specify) _____ |
| ___ | ___ | | Mental Illness |
| ___ | ___ | | Mental Retardation |
| ___ | ___ | | Crisis Intervention |
| ___ | ___ | | Critical Care Nursing (specify) ___ |
| ___ | ___ | | Physical Assessment Techniques |
| ___ | ___ | | Operating Room Nursing (specify) _____ |

## Exhibit 4-1 continued

**NURSING ISSUES AND CONCEPTS**

___ ___ ___ Enviromental Health
___ ___ ___ Primary Health Care
___ ___ ___ Pain
___ ___ ___ Body Image
___ ___ ___ Sensory Deprivation
___ ___ ___ Counseling Techniques
___ ___ ___ Observation & Communication Skills
___ ___ ___ Interpersonal Relations
___ ___ ___ Group Process
___ ___ ___ Nutrition
___ ___ ___ Rehabilitation
___ ___ ___ Accident and Disease Prevention
___ ___ ___ Behavior Modification
___ ___ ___ Change Theories
___ ___ ___ Political Power
___ ___ ___ Legislation

___ ___ ___ Nursing Process
___ ___ ___ Nursing Audit

___ ___ ___ Standards of Practice
___ ___ ___ Patient Teaching
___ ___ ___ Quality Assurance
___ ___ ___ Nursing Research
___ ___ ___ Certification
___ ___ ___ Peer Review
___ ___ ___ Competence in Practice

**SOCIAL ISSUES**

___ ___ ___ Sustance Abuse · Drugs & Alcohol
___ ___ ___ Suicide
___ ___ ___ Venereal Disease
___ ___ ___ Abortion
___ ___ ___ Battered Persons
___ ___ ___ Bio·Ethics
___ ___ ___ Legal Aspects
___ ___ ___ Rape

**PERSONAL BELIEFS AND VALUES**

___ ___ ___ Assertiveness
___ ___ ___ Death and Dying
___ ___ ___ Sexuality
___ ___ ___ Values Clarification

**NURSING ADMINISTRATION**

___ ___ ___ Business Administration
___ ___ ___ Innovations
___ ___ ___ Legislation
___ ___ ___ Human Relations
___ ___ ___ Administrative Theory
___ ___ ___ Evaluation of Nursing Outcomes
___ ___ ___ Leadership Theories

**NURSING EDUCATION**

___ ___ ___ Principles of Adult Education
___ ___ ___ Teaching/Learning Strategies
___ ___ ___ Evaluation
___ ___ ___ Curriculum Development

Please list any additional content or subject matter areas in which you would be interested that are not listed above.

Please make any comments you care to:

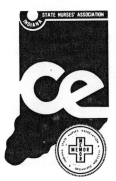

Dear ISNA Member:

The ISNA Board of Directors recently approved a plan to implement the continuing education provider component within the Council on Continuing Education by January 1, 1979. A goal of this plan is to have ISNA become an ANA approved provider by the 1979 ISNA Convention. In order to assume the provider role, the Council on Continuing Education is interested in determining your continuing education needs as an Association member.

The colleges/universities serving as Regional Centers for the Indiana Statewide Program for Continuing Education in Nursing (ISPCEN) are continuing to provide educational opportunities for registered nurses in many rural and urban areas in Indiana. The Council on Continuing Education plans to supplement these existing offerings to further meet your continuing education needs.

This survey will provide information about the continuing education needs of the ISNA membership. The survey results will be used for determining which continuing education provider is most able to meet the identified continuing education needs. The survey results will also be published in the ISNA Bulletin.

**Do not** put your name on the survey form so that your responses will be anonymous. Please complete this survey and return it by Friday, July 14, 1978 to:

Council on Continuing Education
Indiana State Nurses' Association
3231 N. Meridian, Suite 53
Indianapolis, Indiana 46208

*Source:* Reprinted by permission of Council on Continuing Education, Indiana State Nurses' Association, Indianapolis, ©1978.

**Exhibit 4-2** Example of a More Specific Questionnaire: Orthopedic Conditions Need Assessment Survey Form

ISPCEN – REGION II

(for office use only)

Check most appropriate

**1 – 2 I work at:**

_____ 1 a. Elkhart General Hospital, Elkhart
_____ b. Goshen General Hospital, Goshen
_____ c. Healthwin, South Bend
_____ d. Memorial Hospital, South Bend
_____ e. Murphy Medical Center, Warsaw

_____ 2 a. Osteopathic Hospital, South Bend
_____ b. Parkview Hospital, Plymouth
_____ c. St. Joseph Hospital, Mishawaka
_____ d. St. Joseph Hospital, South Bend
_____ e. Other (specify) _____

**3 – 4 I work on one of the following type of nursing areas:**

_____ 3 a. Emergency Department
_____ b. ICU (Special Care)
_____ c. Medical–Surgical (with Orthopedics)
_____ d. OR – RR

_____ 4 a. Orthopedics
_____ b. Pediatrics
_____ c. Other (specify) _____

**5. I am a** _____ RN _____ LPN _____ Other (specify) _____

**6. I work the following number of hours per week.**

_____ a. 40 or more
_____ b. 39 – 30
_____ c. 29 – 20

_____ d. 19 – 10
_____ e. 9 or less

**7. I have worked in orthopedic nursing.**

_____ a. less than 3 months
_____ b. 4 to 11 months
_____ c. 1 to 3 years

_____ d. 4 to 6 years
_____ e. over 6 years

**8. I have attended inservice programs or workshops in orthopedic nursing during the past two (2) years (1973–1974).**

_____ a. yes _____ b. No _____ c. uncertain _____ presently enrolled in course this year (1975)

**9. If "yes" in #8 indicate the content or topics covered** _____

_____

10. My needs or interests in attending a workshop on orthopedics would be rated as: (mark an X anywhere on scale).

| High | Low |
|---|---|

CIRCLE the most appropriate response according to your needs for an orthopedic workshop (e.g. 4 3 2 1 0 )

4 – I am highly interested
3 – I am interested

2 – I am somewhat interested
1 – I have no opinion or don't know

0 – I have no interest

CIRCLE each item according to the above scale:

11. 4 3 2 1 0 Air embolism
12. 4 3 2 1 0 Amputation & disarticulation of lower extremities
13. 4 3 2 1 0 Amputation & disarticulation of upper extremities
14. 4 3 2 1 0 Ankylosis of joint
15. 4 3 2 1 0 Arthritis

16. 4 3 2 1 0 Arthritis – adult rheumatoid
17. 4 3 2 1 0 Arthritis – juvenile rheumatoid
18. 4 3 2 1 0 Arthrotomy
19. 4 3 2 1 0 Arthroplasty of knee
20. 4 3 2 1 0 Bunion and bunionette

21. 4 3 2 1 0 Body image (self concept)
22. 4 3 2 1 0 Cast care
23. 4 3 2 1 0 Cervicle displacement
24. 4 3 2 1 0 Circulatory impairment
25. 4 3 2 1 0 Closed reduction with internal reduction

26. 4 3 2 1 0 Closed reduction without internal fixation
27. 4 3 2 1 0 Contusion and crushing with intact skin
28. 4 3 2 1 0 Curvature of spine
29. 4 3 2 1 0 Dislocation without fracture
30. 4 3 2 1 0 Disorders of sacroiliiac joint

**Exhibit 4-2** continued

31. 4 3 2 1 0 Excision of intervertebral disc
32. 4 3 2 1 0 Excision of semilunar cartilage of knee
33. 4 3 2 1 0 Fat embolism
34. 4 3 2 1 0 Fracture of facial
35. 4 3 2 1 0 Fracture of lower limb

41. 4 3 2 1 0 Fracture of vertebra without spinal cord involvement
42. 4 3 2 1 0 Hallux Valgus – Hammer toe
43. 4 3 2 1 0 Hemorrhage – hypovolemic shock
44. 4 3 2 1 0 Hypertrophic Spondylitis
45. 4 3 2 1 0 Internal derangement of joints

51. 4 3 2 1 0 Musculoskeletal deformities
52. 4 3 2 1 0 Musculoskeletal injuries
53. 4 3 2 1 0 Neoplasms of bone
54. 4 3 2 1 0 Neoplasms – musculoskeletal
55. 4 3 2 1 0 Nerve damage

61. 4 3 2 1 0 Open reduction with fixation
62. 4 3 2 1 0 Open reduction without fixation
63. 4 3 2 1 0 Pagets
64. 4 3 2 1 0 Physiology of Immobilization
65. 4 3 2 1 0 Prosthetic devices

71. 4 3 2 1 0 Torticollis
72. 4 3 2 1 0 Total hip replacement
73. 4 3 2 1 0 Total knee replacement
74. 4 3 2 1 0 Total phalange and elbow replacement
75. 4 3 2 1 0 Traction

36. 4 3 2 1 0 Fracture of upper limb
37. 4 3 2 1 0 Fracture of pelvis
38. 4 3 2 1 0 Fracture of ribs
39. 4 3 2 1 0 Fracture of skull
40. 4 3 2 1 0 Fracture of vertebra with spinal cord involvement

46. 4 3 2 1 0 Injury to nerves
47. 4 3 2 1 0 Juvenile osteochondosis
48. 4 3 2 1 0 Lacerations and open wound of limbs
49. 4 3 2 1 0 Lumbarsacral displacement
50. 4 3 2 1 0 Muscle, tendon, fascia – Diseases of

56. 4 3 2 1 0 Operations on muscle, tendon and bursa – hand
57. 4 3 2 1 0 Operations on other muscles, tendons, fascia and bursa
58. 4 3 2 1 0 Osteoarthritis
59. 4 3 2 1 0 Osteomyelitis
60. 4 3 2 1 0 Osteoporosis

66. 4 3 2 1 0 Psychological Aspects of long term care
67. 4 3 2 1 0 Psychological Aspects of Sudden Trauma
68. 4 3 2 1 0 Skin Care
69. 4 3 2 1 0 Spinal fusion
70. 4 3 2 1 0 Sprains and strains of joints – adjacent muscles

76. 4 3 2 1 0 Traumatic anuria
77. 4 3 2 1 0 Traumatic shock
78. 4 3 2 1 0 Synovitis, bursitis and tenosynovitis
79. 4 3 2 1 0 Vertebrogenic Pain Syndrome
80. 4 3 2 1 0 Volkman's ischemic contracture

QUESTIONS

81. What other orthopedic conditions would you like included in a workshop? _____

82. What other general condition would you like included in a workshop? _____

*Source:* Reprinted by permission of Region II of the Indiana Statewide Plan for Continuing Education in Nursing, Indianapolis, ©1975.

## Interviews

The interview method of needs assessment can be used alone or in conjunction with other approaches. The data are most valid and reliable when only one individual conducts all of the interviews. This is not always possible, however, so standardized forms can be designed so that all interviewers will be asking the same questions. Role-playing training using sample interviews is helpful in ensuring a standardized approach. Interviewing is expensive in terms of time expended, but if used in conjunction with a survey will more than make up for its cost by the value of the information gathered. Interviews can help pinpoint information not obtained from a survey and can clarify ambiguous responses.

It is not necessary to interview all the members of a target population; a small sample can be chosen that is representative of the larger group. The findings from this sample then can be generalized to the larger group if the individuals are chosen carefully to be truly representative of the larger population.

Interviews allow the respondent to express opinions, feelings, and attitudes more freely than is possible with a questionnaire. The interviewer also can give as well as receive information, so that an opportunity exists to present material about the program. However, interviews can make the respondent feel uncomfortable and on the spot. Data collected in an interview can be difficult to quantify and report.

A modified version of an interview can be a telephone survey of a small number of members of the potential audience. This method is useful when validating the need for an educational offering or for specifying its content. This method is quick and relatively inexpensive, unless there are delays because individuals are not available by phone.

## Observation

Observation is an effective method of needs assessment, particularly when used in conjunction with other systems. The observations can be by the continuing education staff or anyone else in a position to perform the function. For example, in a hospital, a nursing supervisor is in an excellent position to observe personnel on the unit and perhaps identify learning needs from those observations. Once again, a standardized observation guide will assist in the tabulation of the data.

One difficulty with observation is that individuals often do not know what they see. For example, they may be unable to determine whether a nurse completed a procedure poorly because she hadn't learned how to do it properly, or for other reasons such as being rushed, or not feeling it was important. In such instances, observation combined with an interview would clarify the result.

## Group Discussion

Learning needs of adults can be identified in group discussions. Members of the potential audience can be assembled for this purpose, or time can be set aside during regular meetings of target groups on other matters. In the group discussion method, a staff person serves as a resource person to help the members understand the task at hand—identifying learning needs. The resource person should be prepared with a set of questions to help the group focus on the task, such as "What do registered nurses on your nursing units need to learn?" "What educational activity would be of most benefit to the personnel of your department?" and so on. The resource person facilitates the discussion and aids the group members in expressing learning needs clearly so that the resultant data will be useful in program planning. A recorder for the data generated is essential. Large sheets of newsprint on which to record the group's ideas also serve, when hung on the walls, to keep the group in touch with the needs identified and as a catalyst for the generation of ideas on additional needs.

The discussion technique of needs assessment also can be used on a more informal basis. At the conclusion of an activity, for example, if time permits the participants can be asked to form small groups. Each of these groups is asked to identify one to three areas of need for future workshops or courses. Finally, these groups meet to exchange results or the data can be collected by the workshop facilitator.

## Advisory Committees

Advisory groups can be invaluable in assessing the needs of the groups they represent. While many of these may be ascribed needs, it is easy to use telephone interviews to validate that those are felt needs of the target audience. The advisory committee members may collect the validating data themselves.

## Resources

Adults' learning needs can be assessed from a systematic review of the literature for a specific profession. Resource persons who are experts in a particular field can identify trends or future directions in that area that can provide clues about potential learning needs of the individuals in the specialty.

Records and reports can provide clues; an excellent example is the patient/ client charts that show evidence of learning needs through the audit process. Research or evaluative activities in the continuing education department also can provide clues to potential needs.

## Individual Assessment

The individual learner is an excellent source for the identification of educational needs. Many adults may lack experience in identifying their learning needs, so that assistance may be necessary before they can specify their needs with some degree of precision. Individual interviews and counseling sessions will provide information useful to the program planner and will motivate the persons to attend the activities that were planned on the basis of their specific needs.

One of the most valuable means for discovering needs on an individual basis is to develop a competency model.[1] In building such a model, the nurse first identifies the competencies necessary for a particular activity. These can be discerned from the person's job description. These competencies are defined in small units consisting of only a single behavior each and are stated as specifically as possible. The continuing education staff acts as a facilitator in helping individuals build their competency models.

Once the appropriate capabilities are refined so that they are as specific and complete as possible, the next step is for the individuals to determine their own levels of competency with regard to each of the elements. This can be done in graph form to illustrate visually the gap between the individual's present level of competency and the desired level. The nurses thus become aware of where they stand in comparison with where they want to be (or should be). Awareness of this gap can be a strong motivator for the individuals to attend appropriate educational activities in order to reduce the gap as rapidly as possible.

The staff have assisted the individuals in identifying their own learning needs, perhaps for the first time. That responsibility now extends to planning and providing the needed educational activities to allow the individuals to close the gap between what is and what should be. The program staff also can help in referring individuals to where they can participate in needed courses or workshops.

As a part of this process, if the individuals are comfortable enough, their peers or supervisor can rate them on the competency model. This can be done apart from or together with the individuals, as desired. They then can further define learning needs as perceived by others with whom these nurses work.

At the end of a time span determined by the continuing education staff in consultation with the individual, the competency model should be regraphed to ascertain improvement as well as areas that still need help. This step is both an evaluation process and a further needs assessment.

Competency models also can be developed by groups. The elements that comprise competency in a certain field are defined in group discussion and are agreed upon by all members of the group. Individuals then rate themselves on the graph in terms of their own competencies. Peer graphing can be done if everyone is comfortable with that process and, of course, if everyone knows each other well enough to permit it.

A final stage in group development of competency models can be the identification of courses with which to close the gap between where individuals are and where they wish to be. The members of a homogeneous group are likely to be able to share experiences and resources that will help each other and provide much information of future value to the program planner. In addition to providing the same motivational force as an individually built competency model, a group-developed model provides support for the members in assessing their own abilities and in locating educational resources to improve them. Of course, the group members should be involved in the evaluation process and in the identification of additional needs at a higher level of competency after a specified time has passed. The development of competency models through the group process can be a continuing method of needs assessment.

## USE OF NEEDS ASSESSMENT DATA

Once the data obtained by any or all of these needs assessment methods have been collected, they must be tabulated into meaningful form. The data from forced-choice questionnaires can be tabulated by use of simple frequency counts or percentages of respondents who indicated a need for a particular type of content. Responses to open-ended survey forms can be categorized under several headings or grouped according to the patterns that emerge in the data review. The results of open-ended forms also can be reported verbatim, although this requires considerable time and may not provide information of as much value to the program staff as when the data are organized.

Access to a computer makes data tabulation easier if the survey form was set up initially for such assembly. Transferring data to keypunch cards and then into the computer is a costly process. Survey forms that can be computer scanned and produce a printout of the results are ideal. If a computer is to be used and staff persons are not familiar with it, it is a good idea to work with a computer department staff member to be sure the forms are designed appropriately, otherwise when they are returned, they may have to be tabulated by hand. It also is wise to have established a relationship with the computer staff ahead of time so that its members know what kind of data are wanted and can help interpret the printout.

## Establishing Priorities

Once the survey data have been tabulated, the needs must be prioritized. Priorities can be set in several ways. For example, the staff can decide to plan and implement offerings on topics that most of the respondents indicated were educational needs. Organizational priorities may determine the educational priorities. A telephone survey will permit potential learners to identify priorities, or an advisory committee can help.

## Problems

One major problem with needs survey data is that they often are not used effectively. The data are not overlooked deliberately but may be determined to be of little value for whatever reason; perhaps the sample was too small, or was not representative of the population to be served, or the form yielded unclear data. Data are only as good as the use to which they are put. Nurses who take the time to respond to such requests for information believe that it should be useful, and indeed it should be. Careful construction of a needs survey plan will help ensure that the time and other resources expended are productive.

Another difficulty is that a continuing education staff will initiate a needs survey when the program is established and the data will be the only basis for planning from that time on. Survey data become outdated by changes in the profession and in society at large. An annual comprehensive needs assessment will prevent information from being outdated. Periodic updating of priorities can be accomplished with the assistance of small groups of potential learners to ensure currency of programming.

## PLANNING EDUCATIONAL ACTIVITIES

Once needs have been identified, the next step is translating them into appropriate learning experiences. The program staff have the responsibility of planning educational activities. Lippitt,[2] Professor of Behavioral Science in the School of Government and Business Administration at George Washington University, identifies four roles of the meeting planner:

1. as a presentation specialist
2. as a planner

3. as an information coordinator
4. as a consultant to management

In the role of planner, the staff apply administrative skills in the recruitment, selection, and staffing of the educational planning committee.

## Planning Committee

The planning committee should consist of five to seven persons. A smaller group may not offer the variety of expertise needed to plan effectively; a larger group may be unwieldy to manage. Committee members should include experts in various subjects and in adult education. A representative from the target audience should be included as a "learner" who contributes by providing a different perception of the content needed, the level of the offering, and suggestions for desirable outcomes. The faculty for the course or workshop should be included in the entire planning process, if feasible. The adult education expert can be a member of the program staff.

The staff have the responsibility for setting the initial planning committee meeting; subsequent dates should be set by members. Six weeks generally is ample time to allow for scheduling the first session.

The staff person may wish to preside at the start of the initial meeting and present the needs assessment data and priorities, if established. The rationale for committee selection should be explained. This is a good point for committee members to suggest other appropriate persons to be included, keeping in mind the ideal size for a working group.

The staff person then outlines the planning process, which then begins. The committee chair can be selected before the process starts and can preside over the rest of the meeting. The staff person may choose to chair all committee sessions unless several planning groups are meeting concurrently.

Committee responsibilities should be outlined clearly at the outset. The committee may be involved in the entire planning process. Much depends on the leadership style of the program staff and the time constraints under which the group is functioning. If the need is an immediate one, the staff may have to take over the planning to implement it faster.

Depending on the expertise of the committee members, planning can be rapid. If the staff person does all the work, the committee members have little "ownership" of the workshop or course and so cannot assist with marketing it, nor do they learn about good program planning. A good balance is to have the committee identify the outcomes, with the staff person then polishing them into behaviorally stated, measurable objectives. The committee decides on subject matter based on these objectives, which the staff person can fit into an appropriate time frame. The committee decides on teaching methods and the staff person obtains the instructional resources. If the planning committee identifies the faculty, the staff negotiates and contracts with those experts; if the committee does not, the staff obtains the teachers through the resource file (Chapter 7). The committee decides on the geographic location for the activity and the staff member obtains the facility. The staff person monitors the planning process to be sure it is moving ahead as scheduled.

Minutes of planning committee meetings should be kept on file permanently to document the process and to meet the requirements for approval by various accrediting organizations (see Chapter 10). A checklist can be used to keep the staff aware of the status of each educational activity being planned (Exhibit 4-3). A good method is to put all of the planning checklists into a three-ring notebook so that they are handy and users can see at a glance where any project is in the planning process without leafing through several files.

The environment in which planning committee meetings are conducted should be conducive to working, starting with a room large enough for the group to meet in. Committees need ample supplies of paper and pencils with which to work. Each member should have a copy of the planning model to be used, so the steps in the process can be identified. If a program planning form is used (Exhibit 4-4), each committee member should have a copy. Any reference materials the staff has identified that might be useful in determining the content, methods, or faculty of the proposed course or workshop should be available. A flip chart with an ample supply of newsprint, or a slateboard, is necessary.

The planning committee should be undisturbed during its meeting. If the staff person is unable to avoid interruptions, they should be held to a minimum. Coffee and soft drinks should be provided. Smoking can be permitted or prohibited, depending on the rules of the meeting location or the preference of the group.

The committee should decide on a specific task to accomplish for each session. Between meetings, the material generated at the previous session can be circulated for review and refinement at the next. Committee members can also obtain input from their peers between meetings to refine and improve the program over time.

## The Planning Process

Planning a workshop or course is the organized and systematic process by which an educational experience is shaped into a structured sequence of events within a given time frame.[3] There are several program planning

**Exhibit 4-3** Example of a Planning Checklist

```
                    INDIANA STATE NURSES' ASSOCIATION

                    Educational Offering Planning
                              Check-List
```

| Structural Unit | Check-off |
|---|---|
| Topic | |
| Objectives | |
| Content | |
| Methods | |
| Substantiation of Needs | |
| Evaluation tool | |
| Evaluation Plan | |
| Planning Committee | |
| Facilities | |
| Faculty: | |
|    names | |
|    agreement | |
|    vita | |
| Facilitators: | |
|    names | |
|    agreement | |
|    vita | |
| Budget | |
| Flier | |
| CEU Application | |
| Handouts | |
| Participant Folders | |
| Audio-Visual Equipment | |
| Name tags | |
| Meals | |
| Coffee/Cokes | |
| Other: | |

BEP:ms

*Source:* Reprinted by permission of Indiana State Nurses' Association, Indianapolis, ©1979.

**Exhibit 4-4** Sample Outline Form for Educational Activity

OFFERING OUTLINE

NAME OF OFFERING: Employee Stress Workshop     DATES: 2/26 and 2/27/81

| DAY | TIME | INSTRUCTOR(S) | OBJECTIVE | CONTENT | METHODS | MATERIALS NEEDED |
|---|---|---|---|---|---|---|
| 2/26/81 | 9:00 – 9:30 AM | B. Puetz | | Introduction Participant Objectives | Small Groups | Flip Charts (5) |
| 2/26/81 | 9:30 AM | I. Benz | Define stress State symptoms of stress | What is stress? Signs and symptoms of stress. | Lecturette Brainstorming | Handout: "How Can You Tell If It Is Stress?" |
| 2/26/81 | 10:15 AM | B. Puetz I. Benz | Identify individual stresses. | Stresses on employee as an individual. | Small group exercise. | Group Exercise #1 |

*Source:* Reprinted from *Departmental Operating Manual,* Division of Continuing Studies, Columbus Campus, Indiana University-Purdue University at Indianapolis, ©1977.

models. They vary from the simple to the more complex (Exhibits 4-5 and 4-6). Having a model available will ensure that a committee can make the best use of its time. It is not a shortcut nor a way of prolonging the planning process by using a group when an individual would do. The steps in the model selected should be followed in sequence. Some originality is permitted, of course, since the planners are adults who are planning educational experiences for other adults. The model need not be followed rigidly, but the planners must recognize that it has been tested and found effective in preparing previous courses or workshops. The steps are not the result of a chance arrangement but rather are an organized, meaningful sequence of events. The basic steps in almost any program planning model include seven major elements.

## 1. Determining the Interests or Needs

Earlier in this chapter, ways of determining the needs of the potential participants were described. Basing the educational event on their needs is a critical and essential step in the process but is not a sure guarantee of success. Other factors such as cost, distance, location, and time of the event can affect attendance adversely. Ultimately, however, if each step in the planning process is followed, and if other considerations for success are obtained, the activity will be successful. Events based on guessing about needs will not provide educational experiences based on real requirements.

Planning a course is a long-range effort. Good planning is not done in a short time. Its effects are noticed not only in a successful educational event but also in the personal and professional growth of the committee members. As they develop their knowledge and understanding of program planning, they will be more effective in the application of that process.

## 2. Developing the Topic

The planning committee develops the workshop topic by breaking down the interests or needs into the problem or issue to be covered. For example, if oncology nursing is identified by nurses who completed a need assessment questionnaire, then the committee may select nursing care of patients receiving chemotherapy or radiation therapy as the topic.

If the identified need is broad, it sometimes is effective to have the planning committee brainstorm topics that may be covered under such a wide heading. The brainstorming process can be accomplished in five or ten minutes at the beginning of the first committee meeting. In brainstorming, topics are suggested by each committee member and written on the slateboard or newsprint. Discussion of the topics should be postponed until the brainstorming has been finished.

**Exhibit 4-5** Example of a Program Planning Model Process

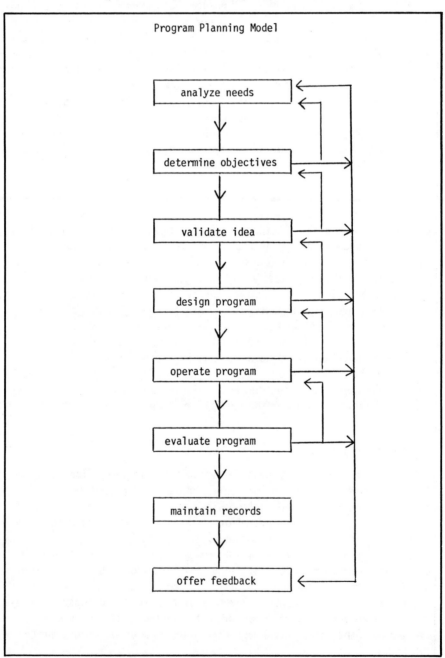

**Exhibit 4-6** Detailed Example of a Planning Model

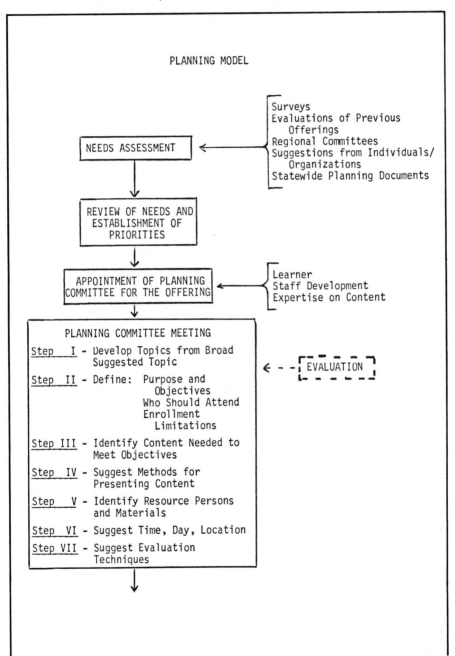

**Exhibit 4-6** continued

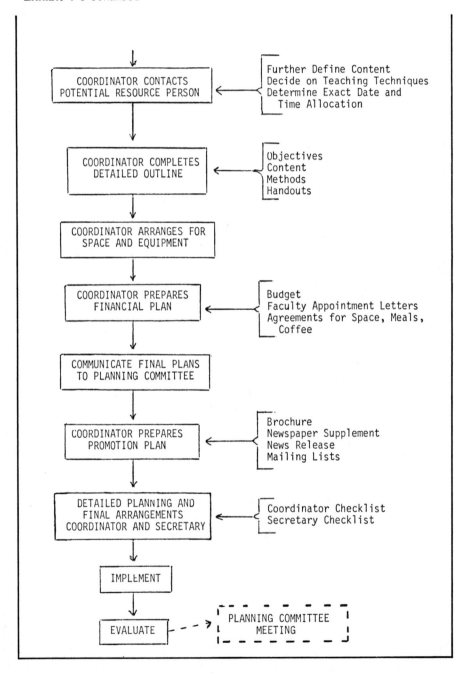

After the ideas are generated, the committee groups them into several larger categories and eliminates those that do not seem appropriate. The breakdown of the subject areas is affected by the background of the planners; if they do not have some familiarity with the topics, they will be unable to determine how to group them. For this, among other reasons, it is helpful to have a member of the potential audience present at each planning committee meeting.

The breakdown of topics may depend on the length of the workshop or course. If most nurses responding to the questionnaire prefer a one-day program, that must be kept in mind so that the group does not identify more topics than can be covered adequately in that time. The committee instead may propose covering the identified subjects in a series of classes or workshops.

Once a topic has been selected, the committee focuses on how to work it into the title for the activity. A general suggestion is to use simple and down-to-earth titles, avoiding "cute" ones, those that are in vogue because of their current popularity, or those that include jargon that may be comprehensible only to persons in the in-group. For example, a title that is jargon to a nurse in one area of practice may decrease the interest of those from other specialties.

Titles should have some meaning to the professional or personal life of the participants and should offer enough challenge to spark a desire to participate. Titles can be in the form of a question to pique interest. A workshop designed to help psychiatric/mental health nurses identify a problem, its potential solutions, and how to apply them was titled "How to Stay Sane in Insane Places." By contrast the title "Psychiatric Nursing," when applied to the same workshop, does not effectively describe the topic nor particularly interest the nurse learner.

### 3. Setting Objectives

The process of setting objectives often is a problem for planning committees. Many lose interest in the planning process at this point and want to rush on to identify the resources to be used. The continuing education program director must exercise skill in keeping the group on the task and can be of assistance as the panel defines the objectives for the event. While the process of setting objectives is described more fully in Chapter 5, the simple steps described here can be taken by the program staff to help the committee decide.

A list of commonly used words for behavioral objectives can be helpful to planning committee members who are unfamiliar with setting objectives (Exhibit 4-7). The members should be asked what they envision the nurse

**Exhibit 4-7** Example of Words Used in Behavioral Objectives

BEHAVIORAL OBJECTIVES

What the learner will be able to DO if learning has occurred.

In stating behavioral objectives, use words that describe ACTION and that can be OBSERVED and MEASURED.

In other words, "What is the learner DOING when demonstrating that the objective has been achieved?"

| BEHAVIORAL | | NON-BEHAVIORAL | |
|---|---|---|---|
| to write | to identify | to know | to have knowledge of |
| to recite | to conduct | to think | to really understand |
| to find | to express | to learn | to be acquainted with |
| to solve | to explain | to enjoy | to be familiar with |
| to list | to classify | to remember | to sympathize with |
| to state | to select | to perceive | |
| to choose | to construct | to understand | |
| to name | to differentiate | to appreciate | |
| to trace | to demonstrate | to recognize | |
| to adjust | to answer | to be aware of | |
| to match | to locate | to comprehend | |
| to compare | | to increase interest | |
| to contrast | | to develop an appreciation of | |
| | | to grasp the significance of | |
| | | to gain a working knowledge of | |
| | | to develop conceptual thinking | |

1.  Behavioral objectives allow for more appropriate evaluation procedures because the meaning of the objectives is clear.

2.  Behavioral objectives must be measurable while the learners are in the learning situation.

3.  The instructor will be able to better select learning activities since the learner behavior is precisely defined.

1.  These words decribe something that is happening in the learner's head where others can't see it.

2.  It is difficult to measure the achievement of objectives when these words are used.

3.  These words permit a variety of interpretations.

ISPCEN
7/79c

participants will get out of the session or will be able to do as a result of attending the course. Those ideas should be put on the slateboard and then, with an eye toward being able to measure the achievement of these behaviors, the objectives can be refined and written in terms of observable behaviors or outcomes. The staff should assist the committee in writing objectives that are specific, not vague, and that give direction to implementing and evaluating the course or workshop.

## 4. Selecting Resources

The planning process for educational offerings often begins with this step. A resource, such as a film or speaker, will come to the attention of the continuing education staff, which then plans an educational event based on that resource. Many such activities are not successful because they are not based on the needs of the potential audience.

Resources for workshops or courses should be viewed as tools to aid in the effectiveness of the activities. Tools should be selected that are appropriate to the job that must be accomplished; tools do not determine the type of job that will be done.

Obtaining the correct resources is a long-range effort. It takes time to obtain the best faculty persons or to select and preview the audiovisual aids selected by the committee or the faculty. The committee's identification of resources can be facilitated by brainstorming, followed by serious discussion of the merits of each of the types of elements described. At this point in the planning process it may be helpful for the committee to seek advice from a person with some knowledge about resources, such as a librarian or an audiovisual expert.

In using such resource persons, the committee must recognize that the final decision is its responsibility. All too often a planning committee's selection is swayed by such an expert or, as occasionally happens, by a member of the committee itself who has a pet resource. All committee members share responsibility for the effectiveness of the activity. It is the staff's responsibility to tactfully encourage the committee to make its decision on resources in a shared manner. One way to accomplish this is to devote one committee meeting to identifying available resources with the experts present, then deferring decisions on their use until the next session, when only committee members will be there.

## 5. Selecting Teaching Methods

The selection of teaching methodology is discussed in Chapter 6. However, the committee's responsibility in this step of the program planning process is to select the teaching techniques that will do the best job. Creativity is a necessary element for this step. Planning committees tend to select techniques with which they are most familiar. It is then the responsibility of the program staff to identify other techniques the group can discuss and perhaps choose as appropriate. Some committees have selected techniques before they have worked through the previous four steps. Again, the committee should work in an organized fashion through each of the steps.

Another danger is to use a technique preferred by one committee member that may not be appropriate for the activity being planned. Committee members should be encouraged to be creative in combining aspects of several techniques to ensure that the method will be appropriate.

### 6. Developing the Evaluation

The planning committee should assist in the identification of appropriate evaluative techniques. (Evaluation is described in detail in Chapter 9.) The evaluation should be based on the course or workshop objectives. The committee again must be creative in determining evaluation methods. If the program staff have a standardized evaluation form, that can serve as a basis for this step in the planning process. The policies and procedures for a specific program may require the use of this standardized form for each activity it sponsors. The planning committee should not be constrained by that requirement. For example, if observation seems an appropriate technique to evaluate whether a specific objective was met, then observation should be included in addition to the standardized form.

### 7. Outlining Responsibilities

Shared responsibility for planning an educational event also involves the responsibility for its implementation. (Implementation is described in Chapter 8.) However, there remain several tasks for the planning committee before the workshop or course can be held, among them the timetable for the event, the physical arrangements, and the publicity.

Individuals from the planning committee can fulfill these duties and ease the burden on the staff, particularly if several events are being planned at the same time. Sharing the final arrangements also increases the committee members' involvement and ownership of the offering. However, the ultimate responsibility for detailed planning belongs to the continuing education staff (see Chapter 8).

## Financial Planning

The planning committee may or may not be involved in determining the budget for a workshop or course. If it is involved, it should be provided with the budget forms used by the continuing education department. Information on the costs of various components of the activity should be provided as needed so that the committee can calculate the preliminary budget. The final budget, however, is the responsibility of the staff.

If the committee is not involved in determining the budget, it at least should be apprised of financial limitations and of how registration fees are set. The staff should provide a brief explanation of this process.

The committee should be made aware of how the costs for planning affect the budget. If sufficient income must be generated from workshop registration fees to cover reimbursement of planning committee expenses such as travel or meals, the members should know this. If they are offered free admission to the event as compensation for their time and effort, the staff should make them aware of this. Committee members often attend the workshop free but are expected to pay for their meals; they should know these arrangements in advance. Policies for this are helpful.

As planning progresses, it may appear that the event will cost more than expected. The staff should bring this to the attention of the committee immediately during the course of the planning so that decisions to pare down the scope or depth of the offering do not have to be made at the end when it is ready to be implemented.

## Promotion Planning

Planning committee members can be listed in the promotional materials for the workshop they developed. They should be consulted about how they want their names and titles to read. If they are to be introduced or identified to the audience at the event, they should be consulted about how they wish to be presented. They should be aware that this will occur so they can tell the program staff whether they will attend, so the introductions do not come as a surprise—or whether they will not be present. It is a nice gesture to provide nametags with a ribbon identifying the persons as "Planners" so participants can recognize them. In addition to this recognition, the planners often obtain useful feedback about the event from participants if they are so identified.

## Approval Planning

The planning committee also may be involved in preparing the materials to meet the criteria for approval of the continuing education activity being planned. The committee must be familiar with the approval process unless this is identified specifically as the responsibility of the staff. If it is part of the planning process and not a staff duty, committee members may be assigned sections of the approval application to complete, such as writing up the need assessment method and results, describing the purpose of the activity, describing the evaluation method, tools, and use, and other related components. The staff then may assemble all of the materials into the appropriate application form for submission to the approval body. If the staff assumes the responsibility for completing the entire application, it is wise to have one or two members of the planning committee review it before its submission. This avoids any problems later if the project is not approved and also enhances the committee members' feeling of ownership of the activity. The committee should be kept apprised of the fate of the proposal, and the program staff should share the notice of approval (or disapproval) immediately with its members.

## Summary Planning Meeting

The planning committee's responsibility for the continuing education event may not end with its implementation. The committee may meet after the workshop or course has ended to review the participants' evaluation summary. Each committee member should be given a copy of the summary. During this meeting, the entire educational event, process, method, and outcome should be discussed. The resources used, both human and material, should be studied and a decision reached concerning their use in future continuing education activities. Plans can be made for updating or improving the course if it is to be repeated. It may be appropriate to decide at this time whether to schedule a repeat session. Changes made before the repeat offering should be reported to the approval body; the planning committee may assume the responsibility for this or it may be up to the program director.

The information on the evaluation summary on participants' additional learning needs may trigger an interest in planning another educational event, so that at this summary meeting the committee may complete one planning process and begin another. If this summary session is the final planning committee meeting, the staff person should send final letters of thanks to the members for their efforts.

If there is no summary meeting of the planning committee, the staff should send a thank-you letter to each member. Each also should receive a summary of the participants' evaluations of the workshop. The continuing education staff may use a follow-up planning checklist (Exhibit 4-8) to be certain all of these tasks are completed.

**Exhibit 4-8** Example of a Follow-Up Checklist

INDIANA STATE NURSES' ASSOCIATION

Follow-up Educational Offering
Check-List

| Structural Unit | Check-off |
|---|---|
| Participant's Roster | |
| Faculty Payment | |
| Thank you letter | |
| Facilitator's Payment | |
| Facilitator's thank you letter | |
| Balance Budget | |
| Planning Committee | |
| Enrollment Statistics | |
| Complete CEU file | |
| Other | |

*Source:* Reprinted by permission of Indiana State Nurses' Association, Indianapolis, ©1979.

In summary, the planning committee is responsible for the analysis of the learning needs of the audience, the identification of information to meet these needs, and the organization of that information into the design of an educational activity, including the selection of appropriate teaching and evaluative techniques. The committee should be aware that it is the participants' responsibility to learn the material presented and ultimately to apply it in their practice. The responsibility for the success of the event thus is shared. The learning experiences have been constructed in such a way as to correspond as closely as possible to the needs of the participants, but they must adapt and modify the information to make it relevant and applicable to their situation.

---

**NOTES**

1. John D. Engalls, *A Trainer's Guide to Andragogy,* 2d. rev. ed. (Washington, D.C.: U.S. Department of Health, Education, and Welfare, 1973), pp. 31–34.

2. G. Lippitt, "Multiple Roles of the Meeting Planner," *Adult Leadership:* 17:4  (October 1968), pp. 158–189.

3. John McKinley and Robert M. Smith, *Guide to Program Planning* (New York: The Seabury Press, 1957), pp. 1–25.

---

**SUGGESTED READINGS**

Bell, Deanne French. "Assessing Educational Needs: Advantages and Disadvantages of Eighteen Techniques." *Nurse Educator* III:5, pp. 15–21.

Cooper, Signe Skott, and Hornback, May Shiga. *Continuing Nursing Education.* New York: McGraw-Hill Book Co., 1973.

Popiel, Elda S., ed. *Nursing and the Process of Continuing Education,* 2d. rev. ed. St. Louis: C. V. Mosby, 1977.

# Chapter 5

# Objectives and Content

Objectives provide the direction in the planning of any educational program. For many planners, establishing objectives often is the most difficult step in designing the event. Objectives are statements that translate the identified needs and interests into learning goals for the participants.

## OBJECTIVE, GOAL, AND PURPOSE

Some of the confusion in defining objectives is the result of using the terminology—objective, goal, and purpose (aim)— interchangeably. To help continuing education staff members in writing objectives, these terms are defined here for use in planning program activities.

The purpose should state why this educational event is being conducted: what is intended to be accomplished and for whom (the expected participants). The statement can be derived from the identified need that led to the selection of the particular workshop or course being planned. For example:

> This offering is designed to provide an opportunity for nurses working with the aged to learn methods to use in assessing and managing disruptive behavior exhibited by these persons. This offering is particularly related to the aged requiring long-term care in nursing homes or their own homes.

This statement indicates that the event being described is for nurses who work in long-term care facilities (nursing homes, residential extended care facilities) or in community health (home services, Visiting Nurses' Associations). This purpose statement is a guide to the nurse in choosing to attend or not attend. It indicates to the nurse that the content will be related to assessment and management of disruptive behavior. If nurses do not work with the aged, do not visualize this as information they need on the job, or feel competent already in handling disruptive behavior, then this is not a workshop to consider attending. If on the other hand nurses work with the aged, feel a need for additional information about disruptive behavior, or have no experience in dealing with such patients, they would want to evaluate the objectives to determine what they might learn.

Goals are broad statements of the accomplishments expected as a result of the event. Some may refer to these as the overall objectives, which can be defined further as what the learner is expected to be able to do at the completion of the course or workshop.

## OUTCOME OBJECTIVES

In writing the outcome objectives (what the learner is expected to be able to do) the following definitions may be useful for planners:

1. Objective: behavior desired as a result of the learning process
2. Behavior: visible activity displayed by the learner (demonstration, written, verbal)
3. Terminal behavior: behavior the learner is able to demonstrate at the end of the instruction process
4. Criterion: standard or model to evaluate terminal behavior

As emphasized in Chapter 4, it is essential to know for whom the event is being planned and something about the background of the learners.

Over the years, as nursing educators have become more concerned with curriculum building, the process of writing objectives has gone through many changes. Early in the National League for Nursing's accreditation program, nursing programs were required to define what their graduates would be able to do. These objectives usually were stated in very broad terms in four major areas: (1) knowledge, (2) attitude, (3) skills, and (4) responsibility. The process of writing objectives for nursing programs has changed considerably since the late fifties as more has been learned about writing objectives for higher education as well as nursing education. Bloom's *Taxonomy of Educational Objectives*[1] (1956) became a major resource for nursing educators in defining criteria for objectives. The taxonomy provides a classification of educational objectives with a set of general and specific catagories for learning outcomes that can be used in curriculum development, teaching, and testing.

Continuing education in nursing quite naturally built upon the process of writing objectives already used for basic nursing programs. Major emphasis was given to stated objectives. One of the first activities initiated after the establishment of the Indiana Statewide Plan for Continuing Education in

Nursing (ISPCEN) in the early 1970s was the development of the "Continuing Education Individual Offering Criteria."[2] Building on the American Nurses' Association method, ISPCEN established criteria for objectives:

1. Relevance to current nursing practice

   - Do the stated objectives reflect one or more of the purposes?
     —acquire new knowledge and skills
     —update knowledge and skills
     —prepare for reentry into practice
     —make a transition from one area of practice to another
     —acquire greater depth of knowledge and skills in one particular area of nursing
     —implement meaningful change both within the individual's own practice and throughout the health care delivery system
     —assume responsibility for personal and professional development
     —improve the ability of other health care workers to meet the specific needs of the public served by the health agency
     —promote and support innovation and creativity in health services

   - Is clinical experience planned to help the participants effect changes in their nursing practice based upon the application of increased knowledge and/or skills?

2. Needs assessment

   - Is there substantiation of the need for the educational offering?

3. Measurability (behavior)

   - Does the educational offering outline behaviorally stated objectives?

4. Attainment in time allotted—clinical and/or theory

   - Does the educational offering format indicate sufficient time for achieving the desired clinical competencies?
   - Does the educational offering outline reflect consideration of the stated level of participants in its objectives and content?

The importance of the objectives to the overall success of the offering was emphasized further by ISPCEN in the method it established for evaluating continuing education courses or workshops. The rating form sheet used for determining whether the offering meets the established criteria weighs the statement of objectives most heavily (see Chapter 10).

## Why Objectives Are Important

Why are objectives given so much emphasis in continuing education in nursing? First, the objectives reflect the input of the learners in identifying their educational needs or deficits and translate this into expected results. The planning committee lists the educational needs, formulates the priorities, and works toward defining learning outcomes.

Second, the objectives define the content required to achieve the results. Once the objectives have been defined, the content should flow naturally for the planners. Statements of objectives reflect both the behavior change and the subject matter.

Third, the objectives assist the planners in determining the methods to be used to present the subject in a way that will enable the learner to achieve the desired results. For example, if the learner is expected to demonstrate a particular skill, the method chosen for this objective must provide the opportunity to do this. On the other hand, if the objective is related to the acquisition of information, the planners have a number of options in choosing the method to be used.

Fourth, the objectives are guides to the decisions to be made about resources—human and material. In choosing the human resources (speaker, lecturer, facilitator) planners refer to objectives in determining the expertise needed to present the subject. If, for example, the objective specifies an outcome involving a specific surgical procedure, a surgeon may be the best person to present the material necessary for achieving this objective. However, if the outcome desired is a plan of nursing care for the patient who undergoes this surgical procedure, a nurse with expertise in the area is a more likely resource person. Audiovisual or written materials are helpful if the outcome expected is for the learner to make certain observations.

Fifth, the objectives help decide which resource persons to involve. Potential resource persons can determine from the objectives whether they will be able to present the subject material using the method that will lead to the expected outcome. The objectives also serve as a guide to the resource persons in their class preparation.

Sixth, objectives provide the guidelines for the evaluation plan for the educational event. The success or failure of a workshop depends on achieving the objectives. Each objective is stated in terms that allow for the measurement of its achievement.

## Guidelines for Stating Behavioral and Outcome Objectives

The planner is faced next with the problem of stating objectives for the continuing education in nursing event. There are general guidelines for stating behavioral and outcome objectives:

1. Each objective should begin with a verb that describes the behavior to be exhibited by the learner, such as define, explain, describe (all of which could be measured by a written test).
2. Each objective should be stated in terms of the learner, not the person presenting the material or process involved, for example: "the nurse will be able to define the terminology"—not "the instructor will present the definitions."
3. Each objective should state only one expected behavioral reaction. For example, define and describe are two behavioral reactions and should not be used in combination in stating the objective. The learner may be able to define the term myocardial infarction but not be able to describe it.
4. Each objective should involve a single subject. If an objective such as "state five signs and symptoms of cardiac *complications* and nursing *action to be taken*," is stated, the learner may be able to state the five symptoms but not the nursing action. An objective that contains more than one subject makes it difficult to evaluate whether the expected outcome has been achieved.
5. Each objective should be stated clearly so the reader will know what outcome is expected.

## Variations in Stating Objectives

Educational objectives can be stated in many ways: in terms of results expected of students, of what the teacher is to do, or of the instructional process. The instructor must have teacher-centered objectives that define what to do to achieve the desired outcome. However, it is important to avoid confusing the objectives of the teacher with those of the learner. For example, "to demonstrate to the learner how to perform endotracheal intubation" is the teacher's role. This does not identify what the learner will be able to do as a result of this objective. The following points state that as a result of instruction on endotracheal intubation the learner is expected to be able to:

1. describe clinical implications for endotracheal intubation
2. list the equipment necessary to perform this action
3. list in order the steps in inserting the endotracheal tube

4. list precautions to take in inserting the tube
5. describe methods for determining the placement of the tube
6. demonstrate skill in inserting the endotracheal tube in a "Resusci-Annie" (manikin used for practicing cardiopulmonary resuscitation).

These objectives describe the outcomes expected from the learners in the classroom. A clinical component also should be included to provide continuing practice in the clinical situation, which then would be written as a psychomotor objective. However, before the learner can develop the clinical skills, the outcome objectives just described should be achieved. As can be seen from this example, the instructor can achieve the objective once the technique has been demonstrated since the teacher-centered objective does not describe any learning outcome.

Another concern in writing learner objectives in terms of outcomes is not to confuse the *process* with the *product* (outcome). The use of such words as "increases," "gains," or "develops" indicates a process that is a part of learning but not what outcome is expected. How is it determined that the learner has increased to the expected outcome? An objective such as "increases ability to identify the clinical implications for an endotracheal tube" indicates a process, not how the learner will demonstrate this increased ability.

## GENERAL STATEMENTS OF OBJECTIVES

The first step in describing objectives is to define the general elements from which the specific learning outcomes can be extracted. The general factors are stated as outcome objectives but do not define each specific behavior the learner is expected to achieve. They must be written clearly enough to be used as the statement of objectives circulated to learners in the brochure or announcement of the offering.

The general objectives provide a mechanism for grouping the identified needs into more manageable segments and into the taxonomy (classifications) provided by Bloom in 1956 and Krathwohl in 1964.[3] The taxonomy is divided into three parts: (1) the cognitive domain, (2) the affective domain, and (3) the psychomotor domain.

With this classification system, all identified needs that may be met best by providing knowledge, understanding, or thinking skills can be categorized in the cognitive domain. Needs that indicate a lack of appreciation of certain situations, such as a need for a change in attitude, feeling, or emotion fall within the affective domain. When there is the need for learners to develop a motor skill in order to perform a certain activity, such an objective becomes a part of the psychomotor domain.

The cognitive domain consists of six major categories: (1) knowledge, (2) comprehension, (3) application, (4) analysis, (5) synthesis, and (6) evaluation. In this area are grouped all objectives related to the acquisition of knowledge (new or recalled previously learned information), processing it, then using it (application).

The affective domain can be referred to as attitude learning that involves the individuals' feelings, values, and interests. In reviewing objectives for an educational offering, it may be difficult to find any that are stated definitely in the affective domain. Components in the cognitive domain may contain statements that can be translated into affective objectives, such as the way a person receives and applies knowledge. One of the problems in stating objectives in the affective domain is in determining ways to evaluate how the learner has achieved the expected outcome. The time available for many continuing education activities is limited. This decreases the opportunity for the instructor or program staff to determine the behavior change in the attitude learning area.

The psychomotor domain is concerned with the motor skills required to perform certain tasks or procedures.[4] Performance skills play a major role in basic nursing education programs as students are learning the abilities necessary to administer care to patients. Since new skills constantly are required of nurses, the psychomotor domain must be a part of the continuing education program. The nurse learning to insert an intubation tube for the first time, as referred to earlier, must proceed through the same steps as any basic nursing student in learning this skill. Psychomotor objectives must be distinguished from performance objectives, which require only cognitive-type performance. Krathwohl in the *Taxonomy of Educational Objectives, Handbook II: Affective Domain* defined psychomotor objectives as those that "emphasize some muscular or motor skill, some manipulation of materials and objects, or some act which requires a neuromuscular coordination." [5]

## The Hierarchical Arrangement

This classification of objectives is designed in a hierarchical order in each of the domains that allows the learner to move from the simple to the complex in each of the instructional areas. In the cognitive domain, the student (nurse) is expected to progress from the lowest level of a learning outcome in the knowledge category through comprehension, which represents the lowest level of understanding. The student then is expected to demonstrate a higher level of understanding by using or applying the learning. Analysis requires the learner to go beyond the application to breaking down the content and determining relationships of the component parts, then synthesizing these by creating new patterns or structures. Finally, the learner is able to define criteria by which the situation can be measured and can make value judg-ments—evaluation. The cognitive behaviors described in each category are assumed to serve as building blocks for the learner to move to higher levels of complexity.

The affective domain consists of behaviors in five categories ranging from the learner's being willing to receive (or pay attention to), finally, the devel-opment of a value system that characterizes the individual and by which behavioral responses are consistent and predictable:

1. The first level is concerned with getting the learner's attention, holding this attention, and directing it to the instructional situation. The nurse who becomes aware of and pays attention to a situation or condition is at the lowest level of learning in the affective domain.
2. The next level involves the active participation of the student from demonstrating a willingness to becoming actively involved to evidencing enjoyment or satisfaction with this involvement.
3. The next step involves the process of internalization in the development of values. The learner accepts the worth of something, shows a pref-erence for it, and becomes committed to it. Learners' individuality (and recognition of it) plays a key role in their ability to achieve in this category of the affective domain.
4. From this internalization, a system of values is developed. This involves the learner's being able to bring different values together, relating them to each other, resolving conflicts that may exist, and exploring alter-natives to these positions. The result of this is the organization of a person's values into a system.
5. The highest level of learning in the affective domain is reached when learners have achieved a value system that enables them to act consist-ently and requires maximum internalization.

The psychomotor domain utilizes both the cognitive and affective domains and thus is the most difficult to classify. However, the learning outcome in this area also moves from the simple to the complex as the individual acquires the necessary motor skill to perform a certain task or procedure. In continuing education in nursing in the classroom, the individuals begin by learning to perform a task or procedure under the guidance of the instructor, involving imitations of what the teacher has demonstrated. Through trial and error, the learners go through the necessary movements (manipulation) to perform the procedure or task. They continue to practice in order to be able to perform with precision (including coordination) and in the proper sequence until they develop a feeling of confidence in their performance.

At this point the performance is considered mechanized in that the learned response has become habitual. The learners can make the appropriate response to the demands of the situation. Beyond this level of psychomotor learning outcomes, the nursing course is more than likely to include a clinical component that allows learners to develop at a higher level, including becoming proficient and efficient in performing the skill, and to be able to adapt, improvise, and modify the procedure or task to meet the requirements of the conditions involved. The highest level in the psychomotor domain is the ability of the learners to be creative in originating new patterns of performance.

The classification of general objectives into the three domains is useful in determining the possible learning outcomes in planning a continuing education course for nurses. The identified needs can be translated into those that require behavioral changes in the cognitive, affective, and psychomotor domains. The hierarchical arrangement in the different domains is useful in designing a total curriculum for continuing education for nurses as well as individual instructional offerings. However, it is not always possible to classify each and every objective, and attempting to do so may consume more time and effort than is necessary.

The importance of using the classification is to be sure that the expressed need is being addressed with the appropriate learning experience to achieve the desired outcome. For example, if the identified need relates to an attitude change on the part of the nurses, the planning should include a review of the affective domain and the types of experiences needed in achieving results in this domain. By using the classification system, the planners are better able to determine whether the list of objectives is sufficiently comprehensive to respond to the identified needs.

## Specific Learning Objectives

From the general statements, the specific learning objectives can be defined. These statements describe in precise terms what the student will be able to do as a result of the learning. The specific learning objectives are stated as observable behaviors and are definite in their meaning.

The specific learning outcomes or objectives are the guidelines needed in determining the content of the educational activity. The number of specific learning objectives necessary to achieve the general objective will vary according to the complexity of the latter. Planners must make sure the specific objectives are sufficient in number, are relevant to the behavior described in the general goals, and at the same time are manageable and useful. Planners must consider what is reasonable to expect within the time allotted for the course or class.

## Application to an Educational Offering

An example of the application of criteria for objectives, the importance of those goals, and moving from the general to the specific, can be made by relating this to a course or workshop on nursing process. The nursing department has determined a need to improve care planning by including nursing process. This decision may be based on nursing audits that have defined weaknesses in the planning of care. Further assessment of the staff nurses indicates that some have never had any instruction or experience in using nursing process in planning care. Other staff nurses have been taught this as students but have not used it since graduation; in organizing a planning committee it is important to have representatives of both of these groups involved. The need established by the nursing department based on the audit and on the desire to change practice, plus the assessment of staff nurses' knowledge and experience in nursing process, provide evidence of the necessity for the educational activity as stated in the ISPCEN criteria (see Outcome Objectives section at start of this chapter).

Staff nurses on the planning committee with no knowledge or experience with nursing process along with those who have had some instruction and experience in using the process will provide the necessary input from two levels.

The planning committee may decide on two educational offerings based on the two levels of learners represented on the committee and the two levels in the nursing area. To satisfy the ISPCEN criteria, a course must reflect consideration of the level of participants stated in the objectives and content. The objectives need to reflect whether the activity provides for the acquisition of new knowledge and skills or an update. For one part of the nursing staff it will be new material and for another a review and update. Based on the needs assessment and on input from the learners, the decision is made to first plan a basic or beginning level course on nursing process, then determine how it also may meet the needs of nurses already experienced in this process.

## Statement of Purpose

Thus, the objectives will reflect the stated purpose of acquiring new knowledge and skills. A statement of purpose could read:

> To provide an opportunity for all nurses who direct or give nursing care to gain an understanding of the nursing process and its application to nursing care planning in _____ Hospital.

The overall goal has been established by the nursing staff in its request for the course or workshop based on deficits in care planning. The nursing department views the nursing process as a means of improving the quality of care through strengthening the systematic planning method. The goal then is:

> To assure that high-quality nursing care given in X Hospital is systematically planned and administered based on the individualized needs of the patient.

To achieve this goal, nurses who direct or give patient care must have the skill and assume responsibility for providing the instruction so the staff can acquire the requisite knowledge and skill. The nursing department is responsible for establishing the criteria or standards required for the staff to achieve the goal and demonstrate that nursing care planning is being met according to expectations. Some of the criteria established for nursing care planning include:

1. A written plan of nursing care is prepared on admission for each patient.
2. The plan of care is individualized consistently and demonstrates evidence of the involvement of the patient or family.
3. Short-range and long-range goals are established in the nursing care plan.
4. Nursing orders are written.
5. Nursing orders are current.

These standards provide the nursing department with the method for measuring whether the goal is being achieved, the staff development department with the expected performance of participants in the continuing education activity, and each individual with performance expectations in nursing care planning.

## Defining the Outcomes

The planning committee working with the staff development department then must define what the nurse should be able to do as a result of the learning process. The first consideration is the stated purpose of the course, which includes the target group—in this case "all persons who direct or give nursing care in X Hospital." The next decision involves what nurses need to know and what skills they must possess in order to understand the nursing process and its application to care planning according to the standards established by their hospital. Another concern is the value nurses place on such planning; the learners on the committee may provide the cue to the general attitude. The differences in levels of learners can be handled best after the committee has dealt with what knowledge and skills are needed by "*all* nurses who direct or give nursing care." Having nurses on the committee with differing levels of knowledge and experience in nursing process is an advantage in defining objectives since the needs of both levels are more likely to be addressed.

The "idea inventory" or brainstorming technique is a good method to initiate the discussion of objectives. Writing objectives in behavioral terms is a process that creates discomfort in most persons, so this technique provides assurance to planning committee members that their ideas will not be evaluated. Many times members of planning committees have not had previous experience in stating objectives in specific behavioral terms. They are on the planning committees to represent the areas of nursing practice for which the class is being planned rather than to provide the educational expertise. In order to assure the contributions of these persons, it is important to provide an atmosphere in which they do not feel the educators present will evaluate their ability to state objectives.

## General Objectives

The committee begins by stating some overall or general objectives from which specific ones can be developed. The aim is to develop a list of general instructional objectives that will help in defining the specific behavioral outcomes to be attained by the learners.

According to Grolund, these general statements can be started with verbs such as applies, comprehends, knows, understands, and uses. These verbs provide the generality desirable for the overall major objectives.[6] The level of generality should indicate clearly the expected results and enable the planners to define specific types of behavior. General objectives about the nursing process may state that nurses:

1. know the components of nursing process
2. understand how to apply the nursing process in nursing care planning
3. apply the nursing process to nursing care planning

These general objectives provide the planning committee with a road map for further defining specific behaviors that participants should be able to demonstrate. Specific objectives can be generated from the general objectives, such as that nurses:

Know the components of the nursing process

1. define nursing process
2. describe each of the four phases of nursing process
3. define assessment in the nursing process
4. name the two component parts of assessment
5. define the planning stage in nursing process
6. describe three phases of planning
7. define implementation in the nursing process
8. define evaluation in the nursing process

As can be observed, eight specific objectives have been generated from a single general one. All of these specific objectives are related directly to the knowledge base required for nursing process.

Another method planners might use is to state a general objective such as "know basic terms." The committee then could establish specific objectives that relate to the terminology used in the nursing process. For example, nurses should:

Know basic terms in nursing process

1. define assessment in the nursing process
2. define the planning stage in the nursing process
3. define implementation in the nursing process
4. define evaluation in the nursing process
5. relate terms to the four phases of nursing care planning
6. use terms correctly in nursing care planning

These describe the behavior expected of nurses if they have achieved the objectives. When these objectives are checked against the ISPCEN criteria, they do indicate behaviorally stated objectives that are measurable.

## Further Behavioral Objectives

Further development of the general objective "applies the nursing process to nursing care planning" could be delineated in behavioral objectives that would require a clinical component in measuring achievement. The criteria indicate "clinical experience is planned to help participants effect changes in their nursing practice based upon the application of increased knowledge and/or skills." The practice this instruction is designed to change is care planning specifically using the nursing process. According to the general objective, participants are expected to make this application. If this is to be done in the classroom, the objective should indicate a simulated situation, not the real world of the nursing unit or an actual patient case.

Again using the general objective, "apply the nursing process to nursing care planning," specific behaviors expected of the learners can be defined as:

1. use assessment in identifying a patient's nursing care needs
2. write a nursing diagnosis based on assessment

The achievement of these objectives then can be evaluated in the clinical area where each participant is assigned. If this is not possible, a simulated situation may be used in the classroom. Or, both methods may be used to provide the learner with practice in the classroom before applying them on the nursing unit. The objective should state where this application should occur—classroom or nursing unit.

Another way the general objective could be used is to state the specific actions required in the assessment. For example, nurses should:

Apply assessment to nursing care planning

1. use available sources for data collection
2. examine data using a systematic approach
3. analyze data to determine the nursing diagnosis
4. write a nursing diagnosis

In summary, the process of developing general objectives that can be translated into specific behavioral outcomes is based on the defined needs of the learners and is accomplished with their input through their representation on the planning committee. The objectives defined in the planning process will provide the guidelines for developing the content, identifying the teaching methods, determining the resources needed to achieve the stated objectives, and developing a plan for evaluating the education offering—the product of the course.

Once the statements of objectives have been developed, the committee should check them against the general guidelines stated earlier. Questions the committee should address include:

- Does each specific objective begin with a verb that describes the behavior to be exhibited or demonstrated by the learner?

- Are these objectives stated in terms of the learner—not what the instructor will do or what method (process) will be used?

- Does each objective define a single expected outcome?

- Does each objective describe only one subject?

- Is each objective stated clearly so that the reader will know what outcome is expected?

If positive answers can be given to each of these questions, the planning committee is ready to move to the next phase of the process: defining content. (This phase is covered in detail later in this chapter.) However, throughout the process the committee may find it necessary to restate the objectives as the plan of action for the course is identified more clearly. The stated objectives may be unrealistic in terms of the time or resources available.

## USE OF THE TAXONOMIES

The planners of continuing education for nurses will find the taxonomies—cognitive, affective, and psychomotor—most helpful in laying out courses at the level appropriate for the needs of the learner. The arrangement of taxonomies in building from the simple to the complex enables planners to determine the objectives at the appropriate level of simplicity or complexity required for the nurse and the learning outcomes expected.

### A Role in Curriculum Building

The taxonomies can be useful in curriculum building for continuing education in nursing. More emphasis is being given to the need for such programs to develop a planned set of courses sequenced so that the learners can choose those that will best enable them to meet their needs. The learning outcome objectives enable the students to determine the level of content they can expect in the course or class.

By using the taxonomies in translating learners' identified needs or deficits into those that deal with intellectual abilities (cognitive), with expression of feelings, interests, values, and attitudes (affective), and with motor skills (psychomotor), planners can develop objectives for the type of course required. Most planners find the cognitive domain the easiest to understand and deal with in writing objectives. The result is that the affective and psychomotor domains frequently are neglected. However, if the planners are required to categorize the needs or deficits according to the type of instruction required, it is more difficult not to include learning outcome objectives.

In continuing education, offerings are presented so nurses can update or upgrade their skills, learn new concepts in nursing care, take courses so they can enter a new area of practice, and participate in advanced study. As these purposes imply, nurses enrolling in continuing education need courses designed at the appropriate level to satisfy their purposes. The hierarchical approach in stating expected behaviors enables planners to design courses appropriate for the purpose and for the desire of the learner.

## The Cognitive Level Revisited

For example, in planning a course for updating or upgrading nurses, the first step is to review the cognitive domain and determine the categories most appropriate for the desired behavioral changes and the terminology that will express these changes. Knowledge represents the lowest level in the cognitive domain and involves the recall of specifics and universals; of methods and processes; or of patterns, structure, or setting. For nurses who are updating or upgrading their knowledge, the planners would expect them to build on their knowledge base in the subcategories defined by Bloom:[7]

- knowledge of specifics
- knowledge of terminology
- knowledge of specific facts
- knowledge of ways and means to deal with specifics
- knowledge of conventions

Nurses' behaviors might be stated using terms such as defines, distinguishes, recalls, labels, lists, names, states, describes, selects, and identifies.

Planners then look at cognitive behaviors to determine the level of understanding expected. Bloom defines comprehension as the lowest level of understanding, when the individual knows what is being communicated and can make use of the information being provided. The subcategories of comprehension are:

- translation
- interpretation

Behaviors at this level may be stated using terms such as translates, restates, rewrites, communicates, summarizes, interprets, determines, explains, and relates.

A higher level of comprehension is expected in the application category of the cognitive domain. The learner is able to use the material in new situations. Behaviors to be exhibited may be stated using terms such as applies, categorizes, uses, employs, records, charts, plans, prepares, illustrates, and generalizes.

## Use of the Affective Domain

The affective domain for an updating or upgrading course begins again with the lowest level or category necessary in attending to a certain stimulus. According to Krathwohl,[8] the learner is willing to receive certain stimuli or objects. These subcategories are:

- awareness
- willingness to receive
- controlled or selected attention

Behaviors could be described using terms such as listens, accepts, asks, follows, observes, is sensitive to, reports, responds, and replies.

From the level of receiving, the learner progresses to the level of responding or reacting and becomes an active participant in the educational experience. The subcategories are:

- acquiescence in responding
- willingness to respond
- satisfaction in response

Behaviors could be defined in such terms as answers, assists, complies, shares, initiates, and participates.

## The Psychomotor Domain — Yes and No

The psychomotor domain may or may not be included in updating or upgrading courses, depending on whether motor skills are required that the nurse does not already have. If specific new motor skills are needed, then, according to Simpson,[9] the learner would be expected to begin at the level of guided manipulation in the psychomotor domain following a demonstration of the task or procedure. The subcategories of guided manipulation are:

- imitation
- manipulation

Behavior could be stated in terms such as follows, repeats, manipulates, handles, positions, places, and operates.

If the learner is expected to use the motor skill in nursing, the course must provide sufficient practice so the individual can achieve the next level in the hierarchy of the psychomotor domain, which is precision. The outcomes can be stated in terms such as performs in order, performs harmoniously, performs in succession, executes consistently, and responds automatically.

## Complexity and Advanced Study

In comparison with a course or class designed to update or upgrade, one designed for nurses in advanced study in a specific area should be more complex. Again considering the simple-to-complex arrangement of the domain for educational objectives, the planners base decisions about results on the presumption that these nurses have a basic level of theory and practice skills on which to build the more complex learning. For this course, the concentration in the cognitive domain may be in the subcategory of analysis, including the ability to break down material into its component parts and detect the relaticnships among them. Synthesis or the ability to produce wholes from parts, to produce a plan of operation, to derive a set of abstract relations would be an expected outcome.[10] Behaviors or expected results described in terms such as diagrams, differentiates, discriminates, distinguishes, relates, outlines, and infers can be used for analysis. Categorizes, combines, compiles, composes, creates, designs, reconstructs, reorganizes, rearranges, and generates can be stated as expected outcomes in the synthesis category.

For an advanced course or workshop, the educational objectives in the affective and psychomotor domains also would be concentrated in the higher categories. The learner is expected to have achieved proficiency and efficiency in basic skills already and to be able to use these in learning new abilities. However, when new motor skills are being taught, the learner still must proceed from guided manipulation to the development of proficiency and efficiency. If on the other hand new motor skills are not required, the learner may be involved in creating new patterns of performance in the particular field of nursing practice. The categories in the psychomotor domain can include adaptation (improvisations and modifications).[11]

To state the expected outcomes terms such as improvises, adapts, rearranges, modifies, alters, varies, revises, originates, amends, and varies can be used. The category of origination (experimentation and creative manipulation)[12] may be the concentration of an educational offering defined for practitioners in a particular field, including a research or study component. Expected outcomes can be stated using terms such as experiments, tests, tries, examines, invents, designs, creates, and formulates.

The taxonomies for educational development can be useful in stating the expected course results. However, continuing education and staff development programmers should study these taxonomies in order to make the appropriate adaptation to nursing programs. As staffs become more involved in curriculum planning, they will develop more courses or classes for different levels of nursing practice and sequence them so the nurse wishing to move up from very basic continuing education to the most advanced will be able to achieve this progression. The expected results (learning outcome objectives) will be stated with sufficient specificity and clarity that the nurses will be better able to make a choice about the level of the offering they should attend.

## DETERMINING CONTENT

The course or workshop content consists of the topics and subject matter essential for the learner to achieve the stated objectives. Broad topics are identified, then the subtopics or content to be included are specified. The outcome defined in the objective cues the choice of content.

If a subject expert has not been involved before the committee begins to identify content, one should be added. If the instructor has been chosen and if feasible in terms of time and distance, that individual should be included in the planning committee meeting.

The continuing education staff person serves as the committee facilitator. In this role, the individual should be aware of some of the problems a committee can encounter in defining content. The committee may need to be reminded of the level of learner for whom the course is being planned. The content expert or the learner who has been involved in a similar class may push to include material that was used in a previous offering but is not necessary to achieve the objectives of this one. In defining content for a two-day workshop, for example, some committee members may push to include everything they learned in a two-week course. Recognizing the time limitation, they may try to insist a "little bit" be included in a watered-down version.

The experience in planning a 200-hour course for emergency department nurses is a good example of how students want to include everything known about an area even if the time allotted does not allow for adequate instruction or for learning to take place. In the initial phase of the planning for this course, the material to be covered could be equated to a graduate course in medical surgical nursing with some maternal-child health nursing added. The presence of persons experienced in teaching adults—working with emergency department nurses, learners, and content experts—would be essential to the development of a course that could be managed within the time frame, could support the defined objectives, and was based on the principles of how adults learn.

Another problem area is screening out content that might be "good for the learner to know" or "nice to know" but is not essential to the achievement of the objectives. Learners' desire for knowledge and the difficulty in separating real needs from interests requires the facilitator to keep the objectives constantly at the forefront of the discussion of subject matter. For example, in planning a course on the emergency nursing management of a burned patient, it might be interesting to know how this person was treated on a burn unit in a major medical center; however, this offering is designed for nurses who work in emergency departments in hospitals where patients with major burns are transferred out as soon as they are stabilized. The real need of the emergency department nurse is to know what care to give there and how best to prepare a patient for transfer, not the long-range plan for treatment in the burn unit. The primary emphasis is not on the details of care on a long-range basis but the importance of emergency care to the success of the subsequent treatment in the burn unit.

If a nurse from a burn unit is used as the content expert, it is important for that person to be oriented to the purpose of the course, the type of learners, and the expected results. This expert may be able to help learners who want to include material beyond what is necessary to achieve the objectives to understand the other ways that nurses can acquire the information. The expert may offer to provide reference readings, a visit to the unit, or other ways for learners to satisfy their interest. Although it is time consuming to deal with pet areas of content or special interests of planning committee members, it is essential to cope with these as they arise in order to keep the committee functioning as a group.

## Identifying and Sequencing Content

The facilitator or the person on the committee with experience in teaching adults should assume a major role as the panel begins to identify the content and put it into the appropriate sequence. The objectives must be visible to all members of the committee on a slateboard or flip chart. Using the idea inventory or brainstorming technique, the committee can identify material needed for each objective. It is best to have the group identify all the subject matter that might be related to the specific objective before trying to establish priorities and putting the material in the appropriate sequence. Through this technique, many more topics will be identified than can or should be included, but these can be dealt with in the process of establishing priorities and putting the content in sequence. The group can test the content against the objectives and the prospective learners to help accomplish the weeding out process. Other useful resources in testing the content include established standards of care, job standards, or performance criteria. The arrangement of the units should be tested for continuity and unity.

Referring back to the course on nursing process, some examples of how content can be derived can be demonstrated. In the planning for that course, the learners were identified as "those who direct or give nursing care," the criteria for using the nursing process in care planning were established, and the objectives were stated. All of these elements then were used by the committee in determining the content.

Using the general objective "knows the components of the nursing process," each specific objective is reviewed to determine the subject matter or content to be included (Exhibit 5-1).

After establishing content for each objective, the committee analyzes the identified materials to determine the sequence in which they should be presented. In this course, the participants must be introduced to the nursing process before they move to the details of its component parts. The committee might title this content area "Introduction to the Nursing Process" or "Overview of the Nursing Process." All objectives and related content then are sequenced under this overall heading. A part of the introduction is the definition of nursing process, including the importance of its being a systematic, dynamic, and problem-solving approach to planning care. In other words, the content provides information on what the course encompasses.

The next step is to present material on what the course consists of—the four stages of the nursing process. The following area may relate to the rationale for nursing care planning. An objective for this might be "Explain the rationale for using the nursing process in nursing care planning." The content must respond to the reasons the nursing process is used in care planning. The material should include planning individualized care, assistance in setting priorities, systematic communications, continuity of care, coordinating care, and evaluating treatment.

The committee proceeds step by step in sequencing the material to provide continuity and unity. The group then can test the content based on the identified learners, the objectives, and the criteria established for using the nursing process in care planning.

## Reviewing and Refining Objectives and Content

A review of objectives and content may result in the revision or deletion of some elements. For example, in the objectives for the nursing process there are four that require the learner to be able to define the terms used in nursing process—assessment, planning stage, implementation, and evaluation. These may require the same behavior as the single objective that states that the learner is to be able to describe each of the four phases of the nursing process. The planners should determine whether, in describing these four phases, the

---

**Exhibit 5-1** Course Objective and Subject Matter

| OBJECTIVE | CONTENT |
|---|---|
| 1. Define nursing process | • definition of nursing process<br>—systematic approach<br>—dynamic, problem-solving process |
| 2. Describe each of the four phases of the nursing process | • phases of the nursing process:<br>—assessment<br>—planning<br>—implementation<br>—evaluation |
| 3. Define assessment in the nursing process | • definition of assessment in the nursing process |
| 4. Name the two component parts of assessment | • component parts of assessment:<br>—data collection<br>—analysis of data |
| 5. Define the planning stage in the nursing process | • definition of planning in the nursing process |
| 6. Describe the three phases of planning | • phases of planning:<br>—identification of patient priority needs<br>—outline of specific nursing actions<br>—definition of goals for patient care |

learner also will be defining the terms, or whether the individual must define the term at the beginning of each section related to that specific phase. The option may be to rearrange the content and include the definition of terms earlier in the sequence. The facilitator for the planning group needs to help it recognize that options are available. The decision on the statement of expected outcomes and content should be based on the best approach for the targeted learners.

## SUMMARY

Writing the general and specific learning objectives is one of the most important and most difficult tasks performed by continuing education and staff development planners. It is a skill to state outcomes that are appropriate for the level of the learner and are sufficiently specific and clear so that all persons who read them can understand the expectations. Like any other skill, continued practice is needed to improve this one.

Content will flow from the objectives if in the planning process expected learning outcomes are stated clearly. The process of defining the body of information needed to support the educational experience proceeds from the definition of general topics, to the definition of specific subtopics, to sequencing of these topics and subtopics. When this has been completed, the planners review the overall design of the course, including results and content. This is the clarification stage when planners determine whether the design is clear to them and, since they represent the learners, will be clear to the students. This is followed by the stage of refinement during which the planners make necessary alterations in the objectives and content.

---

**NOTES**

1. Benjamin S. Bloom, ed., *Taxonomy of Educational Objectives—Handbook I* (New York: David McKay Company, Inc., 1956).

2. "Continuing Education Individual Offering Criteria," Indiana Statewide Plan for Continuing Education in Nursing (Indianapolis, Ind., 1977).

3. David R. Krathwohl, B. Bloom, and B. Masia, *Taxonomy of Educational Objectives—Handbook II* (New York: David McKay Company, Inc., 1964), p. 7.

4. Elizabeth J. Simpson, "Educational Objectives in the Psychomotor Domain," in *Behavioral Objectives in Curriculum Development* (Englewood Cliffs, N.J.: Educational Publications, Inc., 1971), p. 62.

5. Krathwohl, *Taxonomy*, p. 7.

6. Norman E. Grolund, *Stating Behavioral Objectives for Classroom Instruction* (New York: The Macmillan Company, 1970), p. 10.

7. Bloom, *Taxonomy*, pp. 201–202, 204–205.

8. Krathwohl, *Taxonomy*, pp. 98–138.

9. Simpson, *Psychomotor Domain*, p. 66.

10. Bloom, *Taxonomy*, p. 206.

11. Simpson, *Psychomotor Domain*, p. 66.

12. Simpson, ibid., p. 66.

# Chapter 6

# Selecting Methods

The variety of methods available for presenting continuing educational classes, courses, or workshops provides the planning committee with a number of alternatives in choosing the method to be used for the specific objectives. The committee should focus on what kind of experiences can best help nurses to learn. In some instances, the planning committee may address the methods at the same time the subject matter is being outlined. However, until the committee has decided what it wants (content) it is difficult to determine the format (methods) that might be most helpful.

Again, objectives provide a clue to the most appropriate general methods that can be used. If the objectives are in the cognitive domain, a variety of methods may be used. The most important consideration is the target group involved and what is known about how adults learn. Unfortunately, in most instances this is not the only consideration. Time, place, size of the group, and resources available also affect the decision on methods. However, with creativity, some of these constraints can be overcome. For example, if certain basic information is needed by all participants, the decision should be made as to how this can be done best given the time restrictions, the setting, and the size of the group. Is the information of such nature that it could be put in a handout and distributed to learners before the session with the under-standing that they will be expected to be prepared to use it in the class? It is important that the learners be provided with a short session at the beginning of the class to discuss the content and clarify any questions they might have. A test on the information might be used to determine any misconceptions the learners have. If resources are available, a videotape can be prepared to present the information and scheduled so that all students (nurses) will have an opportunity to view it before the first session. An audiotape supplemented by printed material may be useful.

The most important consideration in determining the methods and mate-rials is what will best support the course objectives. The committee must ask the question: What are the functions to be performed and what approach will best support them? Another important consideration relates to the earlier discussion about how adults learn. Most adults prefer to be involved actively in the learning process, so methods that encourage their active involvement can be helpful.

Adults learn best when a variety of techniques are used, techniques that allow for problem solving and that are group centered. The use of a variety of methods will best support the course structure given the needs of the adult learner. Also, given the differences in adults and in the way they learn, the use of different methods recognizes their individuality and their needs.

In considering methods and materials, several questions need to be asked:

1. Will the method support the type of behavioral change described in the objective?
2. Is the method chosen the simplest approach for achieving the objective?
3. Is the method appropriate for the time allotted?
4. Is the method appropriate for the level of the learner in terms of background knowledge, skills, and attitudes?
5. Are the resources available to support the use of method in terms of space, equipment, and personnel?
6. Will both the instructional staff and the nurses be comfortable with the method chosen?

One approach suggested for selecting methods is based on the type of behavorial change desired to achieve the particular objective. Dr. Malcolm Knowles, a noted adult educator, has developed materials that divide the behavioral changes into such categories as knowledge, understanding, application, skills, and attitudes.[1]

## METHODS FOR USE IN ACQUISITION OF INFORMATION

If the behavioral change is related to knowledge that Knowles describes as "generalizations about experiences, the internationalization of information,"[2] then the method chosen may be self-instruction, where the nurse works more independently and is responsible for certain activities outside the classroom. Examples of self-instruction are the self-study units published in the *American Journal of Nursing.* These programmed instruction units also may be requested as reprints, which makes it possible to incorporate them as a part of a continuing education course to be completed by the nurses before or during the event. These units vary in format but in general present information, then require the nurse to give a written response or select answers from a multiple choice list. The correct response is provided in a screened column. This type of instruction is discussed more under the section on non-traditional approaches to learning later in this chapter.

Programmed instruction units consisting of audiocassettes with printed materials, filmstrips, or slides is another approach. Many such instructional units are available and have been marketed in a wide range of subjects. The units may be used in the classroom or placed in the learning laboratory or other location for the nurses to use as adjuncts to planned courses in class. The continuing education staff should review all materials carefully before purchasing or renting these materials, preferably with a group of learners to determine the appropriateness of the content since many of the units are designed for basic students and may be inappropriate for practicing nurses.

Another consideration is the cost of the packaged materials or, if resources are available, the in-house development of such units. Are these materials applicable to several courses or workshops, or only one? Are they compatible with existing equipment? Is the method simple enough that the learner will not find it difficult to follow the instructions? Are study guides included? Since most of the packaged teaching units are expensive, their purchase should be considered carefully in terms of their cost-effectiveness.

## The Learning Library

Programmed instruction is more useful as an adjunct to other methods if a learning laboratory is available for use by continuing education programs, particularly in the work setting as a part of the staff development department. This increases nurses' access to the materials and provides more flexibility in scheduling their learning time. Even if the learning laboratory in a college or university is available for use by continuing education students, it is not as accessible in terms of location and scheduling for nurses.

As previously discussed, assigned readings are another approach. This has the advantage of being less expensive, particularly since it does not require costly audiovisual materials and equipment. It also is convenient for the nurses since they can prepare assignments at their own convenience. The reading assignments should be stated clearly and indicate the objectives to be achieved. In class, time should be allocated for the nurses to discuss the readings and clarify any areas they did not understand. This discussion of reading assignments with the instructor is referred to by Knowles as "book-based discussion."[3]

## Other Methods Available

Other methods for presenting information (knowledge objectives) are shown in Exhibit 6-1. This *compendium* includes a definition of the technique,

**Exhibit 6-1** Example of Participatory Techniques

COMPENDIUM OF TECHNIQUES
AND
SUB-TECHNIQUES FOR EFFECTIVE PARTICIPATION

TECHNIQUES

THE SPEECH

speaker
X

DEFINITION: A carefully prepared oral presentation
of a subject by a qualified person, which, for productive learning, requires careful planning. Often
used with other techniques because audience has no
opportunity for verbal participation.

X X X X X X X
X X X X X X X
X X X X X X X
audience

PURPOSE FOR WHICH USED: (1) Present information,
identify or clarify problems, and present analysis
of controversial issues, (2) Stimulate and inspire
audience, and encourage further inquiry.

THE FORUM

DEFINITION: A period of open discussion carried on
by members of an entire audience (25 or more)
and 1 or more resource persons, directed by a
moderator. It is generally used to follow other
techniques (speech, panel, symposium, interview,
demonstration, or role-play) giving audience
opportunity to participate. The audience may
comment (to be distinguished from Question-
Answer period when audience is only to ask
questions of the resource person), raise issues,
offer information, as well as ask questions.

resource   moderator
X         X

X X X X X X X
X X X X X X X
X X X X X X X

audience

PURPOSE FOR WHICH USED: (1) Clarify and explore
ideas, (2) attain verbal audience participation,
(3) permit resource perons to speak to audience
needs as they arise.

THE PANEL

DEFINITION: A group of 3 to 6 persons of special
competence in the subject and ability to express
themselves hold a purposeful conversation under
the leadership of a moderator in front of an
audience.

moderator
X
X      X resource
X      X persons

X X X X X X X
X X X X X X X
X X X X X X X

audience

PURPOSE FOR WHICH USED: (1) To identify, explore
and clarify issues and problems, (2) to bring
several points of view and a wide range of informed opinion to an audience, (3) to gain
understanding of component parts of a topic and
(4) to identify advantages and disadvantages of a
course of action.

## Exhibit 6-1 continued

THE COLLOQUY

DEFINITION: A discussion between 2 to 4
resource persons (as in a panel) and some
persons from the audience and a moderator.
The audience representatives discuss the
topics with the resource persons under
the guidance of the moderator.

PURPOSE FOR WHICH USED: (1) Stimulate interest,
(2) identify, explore, clarify, and solve
issues and problems, (3) present to resource
people the audience level of understanding
topics, (4) allow experts to deal with
audience needs as they arise.

THE SYMPOSIUM

DEFINITION: A series of related speeches by 2 to 5
qualified persons speaking with authority on
different phases of the same or related topics. They
do NOT speak with each other, but under the
direction of the moderator, they make presentations.
A symposium is often used with a panel or forum.

PURPOSE FOR WHICH USED: (1) Present organized
information, showing a wide range of authoritative
opinion about a topic, and setting forth an analysis
of several related aspects of a topic, (2) help
people to see relationships of various aspects of a
topic to the topic as a whole, (3) stimulate
thinking persons with similar backgrounds and
interests.

EXPANDING PANEL

DEFINITION: A combination presentation and
discussion in which 6 to 12 persons hold discussion
surrounded on 3 sides by the audience, followed
by an arrangement in which the entire group will
discuss the topic. The moderator chooses when to
close the discussion, they then form into a
large group to discuss. This can be used in groups
from 20 to 40 in number.

PURPOSE FOR WHICH USED: (1) secures active
participation from whole audience, especially
useful in on-going class situation, (2)
stimulates interest, (3) allows relatively large
groups to deal with topics of mutual interest.

**Exhibit 6-1** continued

GROUP DISCUSSION

DEFINITION: When engaged in by trained persons under trained leadership, group discussion is a purposeful conversation in which participants explore, teach, and learn about a topic of mutual interest.  Groups usually number from 6 to 20.

PURPOSE FOR WHICH USED:  (1) To identify, explore, learn about and solve problems and topics of mutual interest in which each participant is both teacher and learner, (2) to achieve maximum participation and encourage growth of all participants.

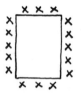

X observer

---

ROLE-PLAYING

DEFINITION:  A spontaneous acting out (without script) of a situation, condition, or circumstances by selected members of a learning group which emphasizes relationships between people and portrays typical attitudes.  Following the role-play, the learning group discusses, interprets and analyzes the action which took place.  The emotional impact is greater through role-playing than reading or hearing about a situation, and sets a frame of mind for self examination.

PURPOSE FOR WHICH USED:  (1) Dramatically illustrate interpersonal problems, (2) gain insight into other's feelings, (3) discover how audience members react under certain conditions, (4) develop skill in problem solving and diagnosis, and (5) help audience members gain insight into their own behavior and attitudes.

role - players
x^x  x
   x
x x x x x x x
x x x x x x x
x x x x x x x
audience

---

THE INTERVIEW

DEFINITION:  A 5 to 30 minute presentation in which an interviewer systematically questions and explores various aspects of a topic with 1 or 2 resource persons before an audience.  The resource persons know in advance the nature of the questions to come.

PURPOSE FOR WHICH USED:  (1) To present information informally, (2) to provide, through the interviewers, a bridge between the audience and the resource persons, (3) to explore and analyze problems, clarify issues, stimulate interest in topic, and (4) to gain impressions from an authority on experience held in common with the audience.

resource
persons  x      interviewer
         x      x

x x x x  x x x
x x x x  x x x
x x x x  x x x

**Exhibit 6-1** continued

SUB-TECHNIQUES

A sub-technique is like a technique, but it is used for a shorter period of time and is used to modify or adapt a technique to the requirements of a particular learning situation. A sub-technique cannot stand alone.

BUZZ SESSION

DEFINITION: An audience divided up into small groups (about 6 members per group) to discuss a topic, or perform a task assigned them (raise several questions about a speech). They meet briefly, usually not more than 10 minutes.

PURPOSE FOR WHICH USED: (1) Gain audience involvement through discussion, (2) identify needs and interest, (3) receive contributions from those who do not speak in larger groups, (4) enable a large group to evaluate a learning experience.

AUDIENCE REACTION TEAM

DEFINITION: 3 to 5 audience representatives who may interrupt the speaker at appropriate times for clarification of obscure points, or to help the speaker treat the needs of those present.

PURPOSE FOR WHICH USED: (1) Ensure that an audience understands a subject which might be difficult to communicate or might be presented "over their heads". This sub-technique may be used with speech, symposium, demonstration or interview, or whenever the audience is too large to permit interruption of the speaker.

IDEA INVENTORY

DEFINITION: This is a spontaneous outpouring of ideas for 5 to 15 minutes on a topic of interest or need, (often called brainstorming). As many ideas as possible are recorded but not discussed during this period. Quantity is preferred over quality. Maximum participation is encouraged because contributions are not evaluated - merely recorded.

PURPOSE FOR WHICH USED: (1) When several alternative ideas are wanted prior to a decision, (2) when many ideas are wanted.

**Exhibit 6-1** continued

SCREENING PANEL

DEFINITION:  3 to 5 persons from the audience discuss
the educational needs of the audience in the presence
of a speaker or resource person so the speaker or
resource person can adjust the presentations they will
make to the needs, interests and level of audience
understanding, or compose their presentation on the
spot.

PURPOSE FOR WHICH USED:  (1)  To be used prior to
presentations through these techniques: interview,
speech, symposium or panel, to help resource persons
or speakers to gain insight into expressed needs and
interests of learning group, (2) to involve
audience and encourage them to express their needs.

*X moderator*

*resource × × audience*
*persons × × × representatives*

*× × × × × × ×*
*× × × × × × ×*
*× × × × × × ×*

*audience*

---

REACTION PANEL

DEFINITION:  2 to 5 persons from the audience or
apecial resource persons  listen to some presentation
(speech, symposium or panel) and then hold a
purposeful conversation in reaction to the
presentation.  This sometimes is followed by a forum.

PURPOSE FOR WHICH USED:  (1)  To stimulate audience
interest, (2)to clarify, solve, evaluate from
audience or authoritative point of view the
presentation.

*moderator*
*X*

*reaction X                X speaker*
*panel  X*
*X*

*× × × × × × ×*
*× × × × × × ×*
*× × × × × × ×*

*audience*

Taken from:  Adult Education Procedures,
            Paul Bergevin, Dwight Morris, and Robert M. Smith.

*Source:* Reprinted with permission from a publication of the Bureau of Studies in Adult Education, Indiana University, Bloomington, Indiana, 1974; derived from *Adult Education Procedures* by Bergevin, Morris, and Smith.

the purpose for which it is used, and a diagram of the physical arrangements of the presenters (faculty) and the students (nurses).

The technique titled "speech" can be equated with a lecture. The term "lecturette" is used for a shorter speech or lecture and usually is followed with another technique such as a forum or by a method of applying the information (behavorial change in understanding) such as case discussion. The speech or lecture can be presented with the speaker in the room, on videotape or audiotape, or by live telecast from another location. The use of a videotape or audiotape has the disadvantage of not providing opportunities for the nurses to have discussions with the lecturer; the third method may or may not provide such opportunities, depending on the talkback capabilities of the television network or facility being used. This approach does give the nurses the opportunity to obtain information from experts in a particular field or specialty that might not be possible otherwise. The instructor or facilitator leads the discussion on the expert's presentation.

## Panel, Colloquy, Symposium, Interview

The panel, colloquy, symposium, and interview also are techniques for presenting information. The panel frequently is misused or is used differently from the description given in the *Compendium*. For example, instead of the *Compendium's* focus on intrapanel discussion, the members sometimes make formal presentations, each with a specific time and topic, with the moderator as introducer and timekeeper. This use of a panel can be effective for presenting information but may produce other problems: holding panelists to their allotted time, defining clear-cut guidelines for each panel member to avoid duplication, and assuring continuity of content.

All too often, the decision to use a panel is made with insufficient preparation. Each panel member should receive clear instructions about the content of his presentation, how this relates to the others, the amount of time allotted for the total presentation and how it is divided among the panelists, the subsequent discussion, and the sequence of appearances. Each panel member should be familiar with the overall objectives of the discussion.

The choice of the moderator is equally important because this person assumes a leadership role in ensuring that the objectives are achieved. The moderator must be skilled in encouraging exchanges of information among panelists and at the same time maintaining sufficient control to ensure that each member participates. The moderator is responsible for ensuring that the intended information is presented and that the panel does not stray from it. Panel members and moderator should meet before the session to review the objectives, discuss the guidelines, and agree on procedures.

However, the method described in the *Compendium* is designed to have the panel members hold a purposeful conversation rather than to make initial presentations, followed by a discussion. This use of the panel provides information and makes it possible to apply it to specific situations as well. In this method, the panel also can address and solve problems, bringing in several points of view.

The symposium is similar to the first description of the panel. The participants make formal presentations but do not hold a discussion. The symposium may be followed by a discussion such as a panel or forum.

The interview described in the *Compendium* also is an informational technique conducted on a more informal basis. One or two resource persons are questioned by an interviewer on a previously agreed upon topic. They agree on the kinds of questions to be asked and the length of the interview. This usually is followed by a discussion.

Another technique, described by Knowles, involves debate. The debate is a good method for presenting material that may be controversial, so distinct differences can be defined and analyzed. Audience participation is limited unless a discussion is to follow the debate or unless the audience is allowed to question the debaters. Again, the moderator should be skilled in this method to ensure that both sides of the issue are presented thoroughly and that there is equal participation by representatives of each side.

## METHODS FOR USE IN APPLICATION

In achieving behavioral outcomes in the area of understanding that Knowles describes as "application of information and generalizations,"[4] a number of audience participation techniques can be used.

### Case Presentation

A most familiar one in nursing is the case presentation, in which the class applies its newly learned information to a patient. This may be initiated by the instructor, who demonstrates how to apply the information to a patient. Each nurse then can emulate the instructor, with a group discussion following.

For example, when teaching nurses who work in the emergency department of a hospital to make a rapid assessment of a patient, the instructor provides the information about how this is done, then presents a simulated situation. The students list, in order of priority, the actions they would take when a patient arrives in the emergency department. After each nurse has completed the process, the actions are assembled on the slateboard or newsprint and prioritized. They then can compare their answers with those of the others in the class. The subsequent group discussion enables the nurses to gain more information and understand the application.

This technique may be varied to have the individual complete the assignment, with a small group then discussing how each person completed the work. The small group then comes to a consensus on the priorities and presents this to the class. Individuals then can compare their responses with those of the class. This is particularly effective in teaching groups about decision making and how individuals and groups can arrive at different decisions.

## Critical Incident Process

The critical incident process is another method for applying class instruction. Some information is presented through printed or audiovisual material. This gives only the most important facts and the learners are responsible for coming up with solutions to the situation.

For example, a videotape is shown of a critical situation in patient care and the nurses must write a description of exactly what occurred. This is a good technique for improving observational skills. For example, the instructor tells the class what should be observed and charted. The videotape is used to demonstrate a critical situation, the learners chart exactly what they observed, and a discussion follows. The videotape then is shown again so the nurses can check their accuracy. This also is effective in instruction about perception and how individuals perceive situations differently.

## Demonstration

In demonstration, the teacher performs a technique or procedure and explains what is being done. Demonstration also can be presented through audiovisual media. The teacher obviously must be thoroughly familiar with the procedure being demonstrated. When the course is being planned, the demonstrations should be included. The room must be arranged so that all learners can see the demonstration and hear the explanations. All equipment and materials should be available. If more than one person is involved in the demonstration, all should be familiar with their responsibilities and be able to work smoothly as a team.

For example, in teaching cardiopulmonary resuscitation to be performed by a team, all members must be able to demonstrate precisely what each person does as well as demonstrate how they are synchronized in working together. The demonstrator(s) provide time for questions. Any parts of the procedure that are not understood must be repeated. For the nurses to be able to apply this technique, they will have to practice or be involved in actual cases, which are discussed later.

## Discussions and Solutions

Problem-solving discussion may be used in the application of knowledge to a problem presented in class. This is similar to the case method. A patient situation is presented for discussion. The nurses first clearly delineate the problems based on the information provided in the situation and in the course material. In their group discussion, the learners identify the problems and seek a solution, using the related information presented by the instructor.

## Colloquy

The colloquy is appropriate for solving problems as well as assisting the instructor and staff facilitator in determining the class level of understanding. Resource persons interact with student representatives in addressing the issues and applying newly learned information to their solution. This method can be used with larger classes to increase the opportunities for active participation of the students.

## The Value of Field Trips

A field trip enables the nurses to observe at first hand a "real" situation, procedure, treatment, or use of equipment. The field trip is preceded by instruction on what the students will see, and the planned educational results are reviewed. The teacher is responsible for leading the field trip and conducting the follow-up discussion of observations made and their application in nursing. A field trip must be planned carefully, with objectives that are understood by the students and the facility being visited. The teacher must determine the number of persons who can be accommodated adequately; the time allocated should be agreed upon with the facility and made clear to the class.

A field trip provides nurses with the opportunity to observe treatment in a referral facility that affects the continuing care to be provided when the patient is returned to the community. Nurses in outpatient community mental health centers can observe treatment in an inpatient unit and relate it to their work.

## Simulation Games

Simulation games can be used in applying newly acquired information and in providing practice in problem solving and decision making. For example, a simulation game might be developed for making a rapid assessment and establishing priorities for the care of a group of patients who all appear in the emergency department at the same time. A brief description of each patient is put on sets of index cards. These cards are distributed to teams of nurses who are to make decisions about the order of priority for care of this group of patients including the reasons for their decisions. Simulation games require high involvment by the nurses. The games must have a defined purpose and objectives that the class understands. They should simulate a real-life situation that is described fully in advance. The nurses' roles and goals are defined clearly. The resources available to them for achieving their goals are identified. The rules for playing the game are established and explained prior to starting the game.

Simulation games create enthusiasm in the learners and provide a good hands-on type of experience. The competition is motivating. They provide intrinsic and prompt feedback to the learners.

The teacher must maintain control of the game, serve as an arbiter in disputes, assist in solving problems that may arise, and make sure the rules are followed. After the game, a discussion is held in which the nurses can discuss their feelings and experiences, the group interactions, and how this all applies to actual situations.

Simulation games can be designed for use in a variety of courses. The design of simulation games is a time-consuming activity that requires creativity. However, it is an excellent method to use in continuing education in nursing to relate the course to the real world. Simulation games should afford the class an enjoyable experience, be simple enough that they will not confuse the students, be easy to administer, require a great deal of decision making by the participants, motivate the nurses to a high level of involvement, and be a valuable educational asset.

## METHODS FOR SKILL LEARNING

The incorporation of new ways of performing a task through practice is what Knowles describes as a behavioral outcome in skills.[5] To perform the skill, the learner must have acquired knowledge and understanding.

The method used most frequently to achieve objectives in the skills area is for the student to practice either in a simulated or actual situation. Sometimes both methods are used, with practice first in the classroom or learning laboratory, then in the actual situation under the guidance of an instructor. For a large number of continuing education classes in nursing, practice in simulated situations is used since arranging for the use of a clinical unit and instructors is difficult. The educational level and the skill to be achieved are the major determinants of what type of practice setting will be needed. For courses that require the learning of clinical skills, a component that provides experience in an actual clinical setting is needed.

In planning a course that provides an opportunity for nurses to acquire clinical skills, the objectives are defined, the resources (clinical facility) to be used are identified, and arrangements are made for instruction. The facility is surveyed to determine whether the needed resources are available. The person in the facility through whom the activity is to be scheduled and coordinated is identified. A written agreement is prepared including the objectives; number of students, days, and hours; and the instructor who is responsible. Agreement also should be reached on the need for malpractice insurance for the nurses attending.

The students should receive instruction about the clinical activity in the facility, including expected results and class hours and dates. They also must receive an orientation on the institution and the area where the activity is to take place. If the activity is to include a number of skills to be learned, the class should be provided with a skills checklist so both students and instructor can track which ones have been covered and which are yet to come.

## The Uses of Role Play

Role play is a method that can be used both for skills practice and for attitude learning. Role play is an unrehearsed, dramatic enactment of a situation or condition that is similar to or can be related to the job. A brief description of the situation is given. Students then are requested to portray specific roles, with emphasis on portraying their own feelings and attitudes naturally without trying to act out or interpret a role. They actually should experience the feelings and reactions to the situation.

The role play is followed by a group discussion in which students who observed the scene describe their feelings as they watched and provide feedback to the participants on their behavior, and both groups analyze the interactions that took place. Those who participated share their feelings in portraying the roles. The teacher then encourages the entire group to apply these observations and feelings to an actual on-the-job situation.

Role play can be threatening to students. The teacher or facilitator must create a climate in which they have a sense of trust. The purpose of the role play and the expected outcomes should be identified clearly. Nurses should be given the opportunity to volunteer. Those who are observing should understand what they are watching and be given guidelines for providing feedback. The teacher should understand the uses and limitations of role play, provide direction, be alert to what is occurring, and be sensitive to the need to stop it when it appears to be threatening to a participant or it has achieved its purpose.

## Videotape and In-Basket

Videotape feedback is one of the most effective methods for skill learning if facilities are available. The students can visualize and evaluate their own performance along with the instructor. The videotape can be stopped as necessary to discuss errors in performance or particularly good techniques.

The in-basket exercise is another technque for experiential learning and is particularly useful in teaching decision making. It combines some elements of case method and role play in presenting information about a particular job situation. The student assumes the role of the person described and responds to the situation and attitudes of those in the situation. The method is particularly appropriate for nurses in management or supervisory positions.

The in-basket exercise requires that the instructor prepare (or use already prepared) materials related to an organization and a position for the student. Each nurse is presented with a packet of materials such as letters, informal notes, telephone messages, and other written communications. The student assumes the role of the person in the organization and reviews the materials, establishes priorities for handling them, makes decisions, and takes action.

The learner is given a time limit for performing the exercise to emphasize the pressure felt by persons in the work situation in dealing with a large volume of materials in a short time. The nurses work independently, which requires them to make decisions on their own. They are required to write their responses, which increases their opportunity to improve communication skills as well as adding to the time pressure.

The in-basket exercise is useful for participants to improve their decision-making skills and their methods of communicating decisions, and to demonstrate how decisions impact on each other in other hospital departments.

The in-basket exercise is followed by group discussions of the decisions made by the participants, who can check their actions against those of others. The discussion provides feedback that will enable the nurses to broaden their thinking about decision making. It also can provide for exploration and more in-depth analysis of decision making.

The in-basket exercise may be used at the beginning of a course or class to get the nurses involved in the activity, or it may be used after the sessions on decision making as a tool for the application of information to the work setting.

## METHODS FOR ATTITUDE LEARNING

"Adoption of new feelings through experiencing greater success with them than with old" is what Knowles describes as behavioral outcomes in attitudes.[6]

A number of the techniques described earlier can be used for learning outcomes in attitudes.

The case method can be used by designing a scenario that describes an incident or situation related to the behavior of an individual or group. The class reads the case study, then discusses it. The teacher encourages the nurses to explore and discuss their feelings and reactions to the situations. The critical incident method can be used in a similar manner in presenting situations that require participants to explore their feelings.

Role play is an effective technique for helping nurses experience how others may think or feel in a certain situation. They often can relate to the roles being portrayed and gain self-understanding in the process. This makes it a useful method for presenting situations requiring an analysis of feelings and attitudes. Simulation games also can be used to achieve behavior changes in attitude.

Structured group exercises that have been developed for use in human relations training are valuable teaching methods for continuing education in nursing, particularly in the affective domain. These exercises focus on the group process with the specific objective for learning and the structure to focus the learning. These exercises provide students with the opportunity to focus on behavior, receive constructive feedback, and process the experience.

The teacher or facilitator chooses a structured experience on the basis of the objectives to be achieved, which are shared with the class. The instructions for the structured experience are provided to each nurse and reviewed and clarified as needed. Needed materials are provided, the setting is arranged appropriately, and the time frame is established. The time allotted is a key element in the success of a structured exercise: the class must be provided with adequate time to achieve the established objectives both in the group activity and in the follow-up processing.

The instructor must be comfortable in handling the structured experience, both in facilitating the group activity and in the ensuing processing of data. The value of the structured exercise rests with the student's being able to integrate the new learning with previous experience.

There are a number of sources for obtaining already developed structured exercises, some of which may be applicable as developed and others may have to be altered to achieve the specific objectives.


## OTHER TECHNIQUES

Some methods described as "subtechniques" in the *Compendium* earlier in this chapter may be considered for use in specific learning situations. These are used for shorter periods of time and in conjunction with other methods.

The buzz session may be a good technique to use early in a course to get the students involved. A specific task may be assigned to small groups to prepare in a short time or a topic may be assigned for discussion. This method can provide for discussion even though the class is large. The buzz group can be used to have the nurses identify their learning needs. The method can be used as an evaluation technique at the end of the session. The buzz session should have a stated purpose that is understood by the students and not used just to vary the methods or as busywork.

The idea inventory, also called brainstorming or freewheeling, is a good method to encourage creativity and encourage participation. The teacher presents a situation from which the class is to identify the problem. The group is instructed on the procedure to be followed, including the time allotted. The purpose is to generate a large number of ideas without concern for their relationship to each other or for their quality; the ideas are not discussed or evaluated. A recorder puts all the ideas on the slateboard or newsprint. At the end of the exercise, the group holds a discussion to evaluate, revise, and refine the ideas.

A questioning period may be scheduled following most presentations. The nurses should be informed of the method to be used in handling their questions. They are provided with the opportunity to clarify the subject, verify that they have understood it, and obtain additional information. Students may address the presenter(s) directly or may be requested to write questions. If questions are to be written, the class is provided with 3" × 5" cards or small pieces of paper before the presentation and instructed to write the questions. Another method, particularly with a large group, is to have students serve as a questioning panel. The written questions are collected and given to the panel, which screens them for duplication and for clarity. The panel members then address the questions to the presenter(s). The questions always should be read aloud if written, or restated if verbal.

The question period is an important part of a course. It should be planned for carefully and sufficient time should be allowed. The learners should be encouraged to ask or submit questions and be assured that none will be treated as silly or stupid.

An audience reaction team is a useful method in planning for large groups of students. This involves a small number of class representatives (three to five) who seek clarification of information being presented or a demonstration being performed. The team members may interrupt at appropriate times to clarify information or points in the demonstration or presentation. This method is useful when the material is complex and the instructor may be presenting it at a level not easily understood by the class.

To increase awareness about what is happening in a learning group, listening and observing groups may be used. The learners may be divided into two groups. One group is involved in an instructional activity, such as a structured experience, while the other group listens and observes what is happening. The groups then can reverse roles so that each individual will have the opportunity to listen and observe. This method is useful in promoting students' listening and observation skills through active participation. The nurses also can become better group members by observing behaviors and activities that support the group process and those that interfere with it.

The class should be instructed on the purpose of the activity and provided with guidelines for use in observing the group. These guidelines should emphasize the outcome desired. For example, if the focus is communication patterns within a group, the guideline should provide methods to be used in observing those patterns.

## SELF-DIRECTED LEARNING

Providing continuing education for nurses in geographically isolated areas is difficult for the sponsor of such instruction. The nontraditional approaches described later may be the most effective methods of providing continuing education for nurses who live far from the location of the program sponsor. In addition, many work in single-nurse situations, such as physicians' offices, industry, school systems, and clinics, so they may be isolated professionally and unable to attend courses or workshops as easily as some of their counterparts. The disadvantages of providing continuing education through traditional methods may preclude their use for these nurses. In addition, as with all adult learners, nurses vary in their motivation, readiness to learn, and style of learning.

Continuing education in the traditional workshop or conference format may not be available or of interest to some nurses. They may engage in learning activities they have designed and implemented. For example, a nurse may want to know more about stress and how to cope with it and may read journal articles, talk with colleagues, and tune in radio or television programs on stress. Such experiences are an effective way to learn. The difficulty lies in their documentation and their approval, particularly in instances where nurses may use self-directed learning activities to meet the continuing education requirement for relicensure to practice in their state.

### Guidelines from the ANA

Accordingly, the American Nurses' Association developed guidelines for the design and approval of self-directed learning activities.[7] The definition of such an activity, according to the ANA, involves a wide variety of educational experiences that the individual initiates. Some self-directed learning may be designed by the individual nurse, such as the one who wanted to learn about stress, but other such activities may be designed by others. For example, a nurse who may want or need to review pharmacology obtains a self-study packet in a learning laboratory at a local college or university school of nursing.

The difference between a self-designed and other-designed activity depends on the extent to which the individual controls the instructional variables. These variables include (1) the identification of the learning needs, (2) the purpose of the activity and its topic, (3) the expected outcome, (4) appropriate educational experiences, (5) educational resources, (6) the environment, time, and pace of learning, (7) evaluation, and (8) the method of documentation.

Some self-directed exercises that may be primarily self-designed are the investigation of a nursing problem, an individual research project, reading on a particular topic, or other independent projects. Activities designed by individuals other than the nurse include correspondence courses, learning packets, programmed instruction, and computer-assisted instruction. Such activities as tours, clinical experience, or work-related projects may be designed by the nurse or by others.

## An Example of Self-Design

In designing such a learning activity, the nurse begins with the identification of educational needs, then determines whether they can be met through a self-designed project. Again, the case of the nurse (let's call her Ms. Anne Jones, R.N.) who wishes to learn more about stress. She may experience increasing stress at work at the same time she becomes aware of greater stress in her colleagues. She determines she needs to learn more about effective ways to cope with stress so she can help herself and others to minimize the effects of this factor on their job performance.

Ms. Jones first must establish her learning priorities. She may know that there is a plethora of information about the subject available, but her focus will be on job-related stress.

A second step is to focus specifically on the project, developing a statement of purpose. The relationship between this activity and others, either past or future, may be helpful in determining the purpose of the current exercise. The relationship between the individual's professional goals and the learning activity should be specified.

In the third step, the individual should specify the outcome of the self-directed study. The objectives or results should be stated in measurable, behavioral terms. (For assistance in the specification of objectives, see Chapter 5.) Ms. Jones may write her behavioral objectives: (1) to define stress,

(2) to state five effects of stress, (3) to list the physiological signs of stress, (4) to list the psychological signs of stress, (5) to identify the sources of stress that exist in the work situation, and (6) to lower on-the-job stress by applying a technique for stress reduction.

A fourth step is to identify resources that will assist in the attainment of the objectives. There are numerous such resources available that can be used alone or in combination. In most instances, the objectives will assist the nurse in selecting appropriate resources. Human resources that can be used include (1) colleagues, both nurses and nonnurses, in the health care professions; (2) educators in nursing and in other fields; (3) family members; and (4) librarians and others. Material resources include (1) audiocassettes, (2) correspondence courses, (3) nursing textbooks and journals, (4) professional literature from fields other than nursing, (5) lay journals, (6) radio, (7) television, (8) telephone, and (9) other similar sources.

## Tracking a Specific Subject

The nurse who wishes to learn about stress may select as human resources her colleagues and a psychologist in the community mental health center. Material resources she selects are nursing journals, items from the psychology literature, and materials from lay magazines that deal with stressful jobs and tips on how to cope with stress.

The nurse next identifies a method for evaluation. In this example, Ms. Jones determines that she will evaluate the effectiveness of her self-designed project by comparing the extent to which her colleagues report she seems able to cope with stress at the conclusion of her course with their analysis of her stress-coping ability before she started the activity. She also will test herself to determine whether she met the stated objectives.

The next step involves some method of documentation. The nurse can write up the learning project, whether or not it is accepted for publication; a colleague could verify that the nurse mastered a clinical skill if that is the focus of the activity; a bibiliography of readings with annotations can be developed; or a case study can be written if the project involves the application of knowledge in a specific clinical situation. The nurse may select an expert in the subject area under study, either a nurse or nonnurse, to serve as reviewer of her documentation efforts. In this case, Ms. Jones chose to write up the project and asked the psychologist to review the work. The paper then could be submitted to her state professional association as an entry in a writing contest the group was sponsoring.

Finally, the nurse should project a time schedule for completion of the self-directed project. This will help keep the nurse on target and help her pace her progress.

As the project is being implemented, there may be a need to revise the objectives or resources. The exposure to a specific area may provoke interest in expanding the scope of the project—or, the reverse, refining the content to cover a narrower area. These changes can be made by the nurse; rigid adherence to the initial plan is not necessary and may not even be appropriate.

## Approval Criteria

Criteria for approval of self-designed activities are suggested by the ANA. This approval may be either before or after the project has been completed. If prior approval is sought, the criteria that must be considered are whether:

- the project is based on the individual's educational needs

- the self-designed activity seems appropriate to meet the identified needs

- the focus of the activity is specific

- the purpose is related to the individual's professional goals and the practice of nursing

- the objectives (expected outcomes) are specific, stated in behaviors, and can reasonably be attained in the proposed time frame

- the resources are identified specifically and will assist in attaining the objectives

- the resource seems appropriate for the level of the person and for the study

- the evaluation method is described and is appropriate for the activity

- the documentation for the project is described

- the amount of time for completion is stated and appears realistic and attainable

The approval body may grant approval for the number of contact or clock hours the individual has identified as necessary for completion of the project. The approval body may request periodic follow-up progress reports or require a report be made on completion of the project, at which time the contact hours will be awarded officially.

If the project has been completed before the request for acceptance, the approval body considers all of the preceding criteria. In addition, it conducts a review to be certain that:

- the content of the project is described completely and accurately

- the content and learning experiences (resources) were consistent with the objectives

- the evaluation has been completed and documents that the objectives were achieved

- the documentation includes the time involved in completion of the self-designed activity

- the number of hours requested was realistic

The purpose of approval for self-directed activities is to provide a uniform way of measuring them similar to that of traditional forms of continuing education (see Chapter 10). Planning and implementing a self-directed project using the steps defined by the ANA will help the nurse develop the activity in an organized fashion and in making it a meaningful educational experience, both personally and professionally.

## NON-TRADITIONAL METHODS

When determining how to present the subject matter, the traditional format of the continuing education course, conference, seminar, or workshop may be selected. However, vast improvements in technology have made other avenues available. Among these are the mass media: radio, television, and newspapers. Technology also has made possible teaching by computers or by telephone. All of these elements are available to the program director who is knowledgeable about their uses and how to have access to them.

There are several advantages in selecting one of the media approaches. These methods expand the size of the potential audience that can be reached. Classroom instruction is limited to small numbers; even if a course is repeated frequently, the number reached still is limited by physical constraints that do not exist when mass media are used. The media can enhance the teaching-learning process and can provide variety beyond the traditional lecture method. In addition, the audience already is familiar with many of the forms of media that can be used in continuing education.

The media approach reaches individuals who might not otherwise attend continuing education courses in the traditional classroom environment. Some of the reluctance to attend such classes may be based on poor educational experiences in the past, cost, or distance to be traveled.

The use of the media may prove more cost-effective than the traditional mode of continuing education delivery. Use of the media must be based on careful thought and consideration of the costs involved in comparison with the anticipated benefits.

## Radio

Radio is one of the older forms of modern mass media. It lacks two advantages of TV: (1) it generally is not national but more local in orientation and (2) it is not visual. For the continuing education program director, however, the first point generally is viewed as an advantage because the audience to be reached by radio usually is local.

Colleges and universities offer courses for academic credit over the air. Radio can be a useful resource for offering nonacademic credit programs. Many of the stations qualified for National Public Radio (NPR) programming are owned by local colleges and universities. These stations can be approached to explore the possibility of using radio for continuing education.

Listening groups can be organized to discuss the radio programs to provide nurses with active involvement in the learning process. Pretests and posttests can be components of the program. This method of communication with the listener allows for monitoring of progress and provides some indication of the size of the audience for the attendance statistics that the program director must collect. Quizzes can be handled in this manner; they can be administered and corrected by mail or combined with a listening group discussion.

The cost of providing continuing education by radio is lower than by television. There are fewer problems associated with transmission, such as poor picture reception in some areas. While most homes have a television set, virtually all have a radio and reception difficulties are less.

## Television

The use of television for continuing education in nursing has been explored in several instances. In 1971, Bolte and Fleming studied the characteristics of nurses who viewed a series on nursing on their home television sets in Kentucky.[8]

Many of the randomly selected nurses who responded to a mailed survey indicated that a large number had heard of the program but had not viewed it. Those who saw it indicated that it was helpful and enhanced their knowledge of nursing. The reasons for not watching the program included difficulty in television reception, the fact that the program was not carried in certain local areas, the nurse was working at the time the program was aired, and similar factors.

Television is quite accessible to most nurses, since most households have at least one set. Television has the advantage of convenience for the nurse, which attending classes in locations other than at home does not. Also, in recent years, videotaping machines with clock timers have been developed; with these, nurses can preset the machines to tape educational programs even when they are not home for later viewing at their convenience. The disadvantages of television are cost and the limited time available for continuing education programming. Production for television is costly; it could be assumed that a professionally produced program is better received by nurses than one that is amateurish.

Access to television for continuing education generally is through a public broadcasting station, although numerous commercial stations make some time available and even produce the programs in cooperation with the professionals and the educators. However, public broadcasting stations do not exist in all areas, so this may affect not only production but also reception. Reception of UHF channels, on which most public stations broadcast, also can pose problems.

Television programs provide one-way communication with the learner, as do those on radio. Active involvement of the learner must be built in as an addition to the television viewing. Methods such as those described for the radio listener also can be used effectively with continuing education programming on television.

Cable television has improved the accessibility of television channels in areas where it is available. The growth of cable television is rapid, so the cost for transmission of educational programs seems likely to decrease. In addition, two-way cable systems, with response consoles in the home, are emerging. The Warner Qube system in Columbus, Ohio, is a prototype.

## Newspaper

A program funded by the National Endowment for the Humanities titled "Courses by Newspaper" (CbN) has been functioning since 1972. The courses are offered in parts and deal with topics such as death and dying, crime, and technology, among others, most of them for academic credit. Their use for continuing education can be modeled after the existing pattern.

Local newspapers may be interested in carrying educational courses and may provide assistance with design and layout once the copy is prepared for them. Courses prepared for use in a newspaper should not be extensive, as there may not be adequate space available on a continuing basis. Readers may lose interest in an extended series of articles. Monitoring the progress of newspaper participants can be done by means of a pretest and posttest or through quizzes. A simple form in the paper at the beginning of the series permits the reader to register for the series.

## Summary on Media Use

None of these three media provide for active involvement of learners without some sort of external augmentation. If students who learn by such means have questions or problems, they cannot obtain answers or have problems resolved immediately, as in a classroom. Human interaction is not a component of continuing education by the media; thus a large part of the desired learning cannot take place. However, there are techniques to permit this human interaction in conjunction with media use—learning groups, for example. The underlying assumption in media use is that this is not an exclusive method; judicious use of media should be based on suitability for the material to be taught and the potential audience for that subject.

## Computers

Thus far in continuing education, computers have been used primarily for data analysis and recordkeeping. Their usefulness for computer-assisted instruction (CAI) is just emerging. Computers used in this way are interactive—that is, they respond to the student in a manner similar to that in programmed instruction: the computer acknowledges a correct or incorrect response; if incorrect, it will review the point with the student until the right answer is made. This is more than the one-way communication using the mass media described earlier, and students tend to be more responsive. The disadvantages of computers involve the cost of producing learning materials and of providing the computer terminals where the students are.

## Telephone

Several areas of the country have explored the telephone as a means of continuing education for nurses. One method is the establishment of a library of tapes on nursing topics that can be used to update or review knowledge. The nurse dials the tape library and requests to hear a specific tape. The answering person inserts the tape in a device that plays it over the telephone. The playback stops automatically when the tape is finished. Access thus is assured to the most recent information on a topic. The tapes carry numbers that are listed in the brochures describing the system. These tape access libraries generally are available 24 hours a day so that the listening can occur at the nurse's convenience.

Once again, however, human interaction is limited; if the nurse has questions or problems with the material on the tape, there is no opportunity to seek clarification. The advantage of such a system is its accessibility to all nurses in the state and the recency of information on the tapes. The disadvantages are the lack of human interaction and the constraints on the kind of information that can be transmitted since hearing is the only sense involved; some things are better seen as well as heard.

The telephone also may be used for continuing education teleconferences. A telephone network is established that provides for a conference call to the facilities that connects them with the originating point. Nurses assemble in rooms equipped with loudspeakers to receive the teleconference call. The presentation is followed by a question and discussion period involving nurses in all the locations.

The teleconference has the advantage of involving the nurses in the educational activity through questions and discussion. They can interact with and learn from each other without having to travel to different locations. The teleconference does require special equipment, and there is, of course, the phone toll charge.

## Programmed Instruction

Programmed instruction was a direct result of the work of B. F. Skinner on operant conditioning. For some students it is a most effective mode of learning. The programmed instruction materials are printed in various forms, the basis for the instruction is presented carefully in sequential steps, and the correct response is noted after each step. Various means of response are possible: words can be filled in or underlined, responses noted as true or false, sentences corrected or otherwise changed, and so on. Programmed instruction gives immediate feedback to the learner about the correctness of the responses. Review usually is necessary if the response is incorrect. Programmed instruction involves much repetition and thus can become boring for some students. The judgment as to whether to use programmed instruction depends primarily on the quality of the materials, how complete they are, how well they cover the topic, how appropriate they are for the level of learner, and how easy it is to follow the accompanying directions.

All of these methods of nontraditional continuing education have their uses. The discriminating continuing education director selects those that will meet the needs of the students on subjects that can be taught best using such approaches.

## NOTES

1. Malcolm Knowles, *The Modern Practice of Adult Education* (New York: Association Press, 1970), p. 294.

2. Ibid., p. 294.

3. Ibid.

4. Ibid.

5. Ibid.

6. Ibid.

7. American Nurses' Association, *Self-Directed Continuing Education in Nursing* (Kansas City, Mo.: American Nurses' Association, 1978), pp. 1–7.

8. I. Bolte and J. Fleming, "A Study of Registered Nurses Who Viewed the PANMED Television Series in Nursing," *The Journal of Continuing Education in Nursing,* September-October 1971, pp. 13–20.

## SUGGESTED READING

Chamberlain, Martin, N., ed. *Providing Continuing Education by Media and Technology: 5* (San Francisco: Jossey-Bass, Inc.), 1980.

# Chapter 7

# Resource Identification

The use of appropriate resources is imperative to ensure the quality and the cost-effectiveness of a continuing education activity. These resources can be classified as human or material (including financial).

## HUMAN RESOURCES

When selecting human resources, it usually is the program planning committee that has the responsibility for identifying the faculty members appropriate for the proposed event. It is helpful if the continuing education department has established a resource file from which an appropriate instructor can be selected. The development of a faculty resource file is a systematic process but should not consume so much time that it loses its value to the program because of its cost.

To develop a faculty resource file, the continuing education program director should decide what instructors—as types and as individuals—are being sought. The instructors should be compatible with the philosophy of the department; that is, they should be comfortable with its concepts of adult education and the teaching-learning process. The department's reputation depends in large part on the effectiveness and general acceptability of the activities it sponsors. Therefore, the faculty must be of the highest caliber to enhance that reputation, rather than to detract from it. It is essential to develop a pool of well-qualified instructors from which to draw rather than making random selections based on the need to present a particular subject.

It is helpful in choosing these individuals to state what will be expected of them—for example, the size of group they will be working with and what their tasks will be (in addition to preparing the content), such as serving on the planning committee, writing objectives, or other administrative work. The department should develop a course description so the instructors can decide whether they indeed are interested in being a part of the faculty resource file. A well-designed set of expectations and qualifications for prospective faculty will allow a better fit between instructor and activity. While an extensive work description for the faculty of a one-day workshop may be impractical, there nevertheless must be a clear definition of what is expected of instructors.

## Selection Criteria

In selecting instructors for a faculty resource file, several criteria are essential. The faculty persons must be continuing learners, otherwise they may not communicate the importance of lifelong learning to the participants in a continuing education offering. Their involvement is not necessarily restricted to their level of formal education. Commitment to or involvement in professional associations, reading professional journals, and participating in continuing education activities other than the ones they are teaching is important. Since a significant message that the instructors will convey is a thirst for continuing to learn, they must be role models for the students.

If instructors are not comfortable in the class environment, there will be a credibility gap between faculty and students. Much of value will be lost if the participants feel the instructors are from the "ivory tower of academia" and far removed from the realities of the situation in which the nurses must practice. This can be offset by having a theoretician and a practitioner "team teach" so that both aspects are covered equally. In continuing education, the emphasis should be on experiential rather than pedagogical expertise, since the faculty works with practicing nurses.

Skill in working with adults is a quality that is essential for the faculty. Because many of the classes are heterogeneous, the faculty must be skilled at presenting the subject for various levels of expertise.

The experiences represented in a typical class provide a vast base upon which the faculty can rest theoretical principles. The learners may require extra assistance in translating a subject into practice immediately. The skillful instructor works to overcome nurses' biases and prejudices because of their experiences, such as "That won't work in my setting," or "Yes, that's a good idea, BUT." Often such resistance occurs when the course or workshop material involves subjects that are uncomfortable for the nurses, such as mental health, substance abuse, death and dying, or human sexuality.

The faculty member must be comfortable with teaching techniques that involve learners' active participation. Most nurses learn through the traditional lecture method and tend to be reluctant to accept other methods as equally valid or effective. If the instructor is uncomfortable leading a small group discussion, then that technique may disintegrate into the "blind leading the blind" and further reinforce its lack of value in the participants' minds.

## The Need for Interpersonal Skills

Working effectively with adults in continuing education requires interpersonal skills based on acceptance of individuals where they are. All participants do not relate to instructors the same way. Many may respond well to a faculty member who is enthusiastic and outgoing, but others may relate better to a more reserved, quieter individual. This should be taken into consideration when reviewing participants' evaluations of their classes. Whatever the instructors' personalities, they must convey genuine concern for their students; this can make the difference between a successful and an unsuccessful course.

The faculty member must be flexible because of the diverse nature of the students. For example, the material prepared by the instructor may be too basic for the class. If the planning committee includes an audience representative, this should not happen, but even in the best planned courses, something can go wrong. The faculty may need to adjust the level of the material on the very day it is being presented. Some other element may go awry, but the instructor cannot come unglued and must carry on without undue stress. If a film tears irreparably, the teacher must cover the subject without it. The teacher must be flexible enough to realize when time should be devoted to discussion of the participants' ideas or problems and when the focus should be returned to the subject of the course or workshop. It is frustrating for participants to spend endless time on one individual's situation, or conversely, not to be permitted to discuss their own problems at all. Flexible instructors can achieve a balance between the two extremes.

Because of the importance of nurses exchanging information and ideas, the in-class time frame does not have to be constructed tightly. Flexible teachers, however, have materials available if there is time to be filled. Parts of the material can be marked for deletion or are optional if time does not permit covering those aspects adequately.

The instructor also must be flexible enough to work with various members of the continuing education program. Depending on the activity, the faculty member may work with the planning committee, the continuing education professional staff, support staff, or other instructors, in addition to the learners (nurses). Some of these persons may have ideas that are not compatible with those of the instructor either in the subject area or in working with adults. Students also may dispute what the teacher says if they disagree with the instructor's viewpoint and disrupt the class. The instructor must focus on the purpose of the activity and not allow differences of opinion to degenerate into serious arguments. Such occurrences should be handled privately at the close of class.

The instructor must be creative. Creative individuals will develop nontraditional ways to help adults learn. They will help the nurses find their own answers instead of being the source of all the knowledge, thereby fostering independent learning.

In summary, the instructor must have knowledge of the subject, skill in using a variety of teaching methods involving active participation of the learners, as well as the personal characteristics of flexibility, ability to relate well to others, ability to communicate, and interest in teaching adults in the continuing education environment. If a specific learning method has been identified by the planning committee, an instructor must be selected who is comfortable with that system. For that and other reasons, it is important to involve the teacher in the planning process wherever feasible.

## How to Find Faculty Members

Identification of potential candidates for a faculty resource file is a continuing process. Names should be added whenever potential instructors are located. Ways of finding faculty members abound. Planning committee members are excellent resources for identifying those with whom they have had contact in previous courses or workshops. Instructors in schools of nursing often are interested in teaching continuing education in addition to their regular employment. Students in graduate nursing programs or in other disciplines may be willing to serve as faculty in their areas of expertise.

Professional publications carry articles by individuals who are potential instructors for the subjects they cover. Fliers and catalogs of other continuing education programs may suggest faculty resources, as well as topics that may be of interest to the nurses in the potential audience. Care must be taken not to become entangled in competition for faculty. Collaborative ventures in which faculty members are shared will be more successful.

Professional associations are sources for potential faculty, as are community sources such as business and industrial firms, other professionals such as physicians and dentists, or officers of voluntary health agencies such as the heart association, and others.

Continuing education staff members also are valuable sources of potential instructors. Because of their involvement in continuing education, they have made contacts with other educators and have participated in activities from which future faculty members can be identified.

Another valuable resource is the teachers who apply to the program planner to take on courses. As the continuing education program grows and establishes a reputation for excellence, more and more such offers will be made. Caution must be exercised, however, and checks on volunteers must be every bit as rigorous as those on faculty members identified in other ways so that the program's quality won't be jeopardized by inadequate choices.

## Screening for the Best

Once potential faculty members have been identified, they must be screened to be sure that only the most qualifed are accepted. The selections should be made on the basis of their ability to relate to adult learners and their knowledge of the subject to be taught. The department staff should check references, such as program directors where the instructors previously served as faculty or who actually observed the individuals in class. Evaluations by participants in previous courses taught by the potential faculty members are useful.

Obviously, all potential instructors must know much more about their subjects than do the students. For example, it is helpful if an instructor is knowledgeable not only about the theory of dialysis but also is familiar with a typical renal dialysis unit in a hospital.

Although most continuing education courses or workshops tend to focus on a specific subject, the instructors also may include material from their studies of areas outside of nursing practice that relate to the class topic. For example, the psychological and sociological effects of renal dialysis should be integrated with information on anatomy/physiology, dialysis technique, and nursing care. However, instructors need not know *everything* about a topic; even possession of total knowledge about a subject does not guarantee that an individual will be a good teacher of adults. Instructors who feel a need to be all-knowing about a subject may be threatened when students seem to know as much as, or more than, they do. Effective teachers use the collective knowledge in the class, enhanced by their own, to help the nurses achieve their educational objectives.

Faculty members not only must be knowledgeable about their subject but also must know how to conduct courses for adults using a variety of teaching methods that involve students' active participation. For example, a teacher who is not skilled in leading group discussions should be assisted by a facilitator who is. Some teachers are used to lecturing only and don't know how to facilitate group discussion. If a physician is to lecture on a new surgical technique, the planning committee can prepare case studies on the nursing care involved so the nurses can apply what they learn to a simulated situation with which they are familiar and, ultimately, to an actual situation. If the students are used as a resource to identify the applicability of the material, the class can be made more relevant to them and have an impact on their subsequent performance.

The instructor can identify helpful resources such as handouts, bibliographies, or audiovisuals, but these materials should not be restricted to those selected by the teacher. Planning committee members have the responsibility of identifying all of the resources necessary for a course or workshop.

In summary, selection of an instructor does not eliminate the responsibility of the planning committee or, ultimately, of the continuing education staff to ensure the effectiveness of the course. The planning committee and staff remain involved until the activity has been implemented and evaluated.

Once faculty members have been selected, current vitae should be requested for the files and for use in the promotional materials. A standardized vita form will permit the same information to be obtained from each person in the faculty resource file (Exhibit 7-1).

Following the activity, participant evaluations should be used to update the faculty resource file. Of course, if these evaluations are unfavorable, a decision must be made whether to keep that person on the faculty. It is helpful for a program staff member or someone from the planning committee to have attended the class so firsthand observations of the teacher's performance can be recorded.

## MATERIAL RESOURCES

Material resources (including financial) are important components in planning and implementing continuing education. In selecting course materials, the planning committee may consider audiovisual or other resources.

### Audiovisual Aids

When audiovisual aids are identified as a material resource, the planning committee must consider first the intended audience. The size of the group will be a determining factor. If it is large, a 16mm film probably will be the most appropriate selection. Audiotapes and videotapes are useful in small groups or by individuals. Slides and overhead transparencies are effective in both small and large groups. Programmed instruction materials are more suitable for individuals, although group discussions can be structured around such aids.

#### Importance of the Physical Environment

The physical environment in which the audiovisual materials are used is important. Films require that the room be darkened. A room without sufficient curtains or window shades is not suitable. Students become frustrated trying to view a film in a lighted room and thus fail to obtain the needed information.

**Exhibit 7-1** Example of a Standardized Vita Form

```
        INDIANA STATEWIDE PLAN FOR CONTINUING EDUCATION IN NURSING

                        VITA SHEET FOR INSTRUCTORS

        Mr.
NAME    Mrs. _____
        Miss      (Last)          (First)         (Middle)        (Maiden)

ADDRESS (Home) _____
                  (Number)         (Street)         (City)         (Zip)

EMPLOYMENT NAME _____


                  (Number)         (Street)         (City)         (Zip)

Responsibilities on Present Position _____

_____

_____

_____


EDUCATIONAL DATA          Institution                 Degree    Major    Year

               _____

               _____

               _____

               _____

PREVIOUS EXPERIENCE _____

_____

_____

_____


AREAS OF INTEREST, SPECIALIZATION OR EXPERTISE IN RELATION TO THIS COURSE _____

_____

_____

_____

_____

_____

_____


No. 2/2-1-74
```

A room need not be totally darkened for videocassettes, since they can be played on a television set. Several sets may be needed if the room is large or the size of the group precludes everyone's being able to view one set. Overhead transparencies require some darkening of the room, but less than for a film.

Audiocassettes can be played in almost any situation. However, if they are used for large groups, provision must be made to plug the tape recorder into the room's public address system rather than rely on the audio capacity of the recorder. Again, if the audiocassette cannot be heard by the entire class, the substance will be lost and the students frustrated.

## Content Should Be Supportive

The content of the audiovisual aid is a concern of the planning committee. The material should enhance that of the class topic. Audiovisual aids that are peripheral to the subject may require so much explanation of their relevance that their value is lost.

The subject may be expressed through sound alone, such as with audiocassettes, or by using both sound and sight. Interviewing and counseling, for example, are taught best with both sound and sight so that the verbal and nonverbal communications are clear enough for the participants to learn appropriate techniques.

## Availability and Previewing

The planning committee also must consider the availability of audiovisual aids. They can be rented, purchased, or borrowed. Renting can be done through college or university audiovisual departments or professional organizations, voluntary health agencies, and publishing companies. Rental policies vary with the organization. It is imperative to check well in advance of the need lest the day of the class arrive and the audiovisual aid is found to be unavailable. Most audiovisual suppliers have catalogs listing rentals, often with provision for previews. Discussion guides and other learning aids associated with the audiovisual material may be available; users should be sure to inquire about them if they are not noted in the catalog.

A preview should be arranged where possible, noting carefully the length of the film or tape, so that an appropriate amount of time can be allotted. One cautionary word about when audiovisual materials should be used: it is not advisable to use such aids, particularly those requiring the room to be darkened, right after lunch—the participants tend to doze off (and so might the instructor).

*To Buy or To Borrow*

It is expensive to purchase audiovisual aids so it should be certain that they will have more than limited usefulness before an investment is made. Catalogs are readily available listing sources where audiovisual aids can be purchased. Again, a preview is helpful in deciding whether to buy. Some companies charge for previewing before purchase, but if the decision is made not to buy it is better to lose the preview fee (usually small) than to be stuck with an audiovisual aid that is not useful.

Borrowing audiovisual aids is an inexpensive means of providing such materials. Public libraries often have such materials available for a nominal charge. Library collections usually are fairly general—that is, not necessarily specific to nursing but, for example, appropriate to teach principles of communication that then can be applied to nursing practice situations through case study or group discussion. Again, a preview is essential to be certain that the aids contain the necessary material. Colleges or universities may have audiocassettes or videocassettes on topics pertinent to their various departments. A psychology department, for example, may have materials on the growth and development of children that would be useful for a pediatric nursing class. Voluntary health agencies often have audiovisual aids that are worth borrowing when they are appropriate for a specific class.

Borrowing audiovisual materials implies that they will be returned in the condition in which they were obtained. If something happens to the material, the renter or borrower must report the damage and assume financial responsibility for repair or replacement. For that reason, it is wise for the program staff to assume personal responsibility for audiovisual aids.

Another consideration when selecting audiovisual aids is the availability of equipment, which also can be purchased, rented, or borrowed. Basic equipment for a continuing education department includes a 16mm projector (preferably automatic threading), an overhead projector for transparencies, and a carousel slide projector.

If purchase is not possible, rental may be the next best option. Many cities have firms that rent equipment of all kinds for educational activities. Delivery in time for the class and pick-up afterward usually are available at a nominal additional charge.

Many hotels and motels will provide audiovisual equipment without charge, along with the room in which to hold the class or workshop. Arrangements must be made well in advance as other groups often are booked in the same hotel at the same time and certain kinds of equipment may be limited in their availability.

Colleges and universities may make equipment available as a service of their audiovisual departments. Again, arrangements must be made well in advance, particularly when the classes are in times of peak demand.

## Other Material Resources

Material resources other than audiovisual aids are useful adjuncts. Bibliographies can be compiled by members of the planning committee. The instructor may have a bibliography prepared; the planning committee may simply review and update it. Bibliographies can be prepared through a college or university librarian if that is a service offered, or through computer searches.

A bibliography can be compiled through a computer search of the two indexes in the Educational Resources Information Center (ERIC), which is a national information system supported by the United States Department of Education and is located in Washington, D.C. The ERIC system collects and disseminates information about research in education.

The computer search of ERIC involves: (1) *Resources in Education* (RIE) and (2) the *Current Index to Journals in Education* (CIJE). *Resources in Education* is a monthly journal that lists research reports by subject, author, and title. Each report has a full citation and an abstract. *Current Index to Journals in Education* is a monthly index of more than 500 journals. Both of these sources also cover related topics such as consumer or environmental education, the handicapped, senior citizens, community development, and minority groups.

The computer printout lists the most recent journal articles from CIJE and the research reports from RIE that match topics selected from an extensive list of descriptors entered into the computer. The first 100 of these citations also include abstracts; abstracts for all citations are available for an additional fee. The computer search of ERIC generally is done for the previous 10 to 15 years. Retrospective searches beyond the previous 10 to 15 years are available at a small additional cost. The reports are available from ERIC either in microfiche or photocopy.

When a request is made for a computer search of ERIC, the printout is received in four to seven days. The price is reasonable—the average cost for both searches (RIE and CIJE) is less than $10. Accessibility is not limited to employees of educational institutions; anyone may request the service where it is available.

A search of literature in health fields is available through the Medical Literature Access and Retrieval System (MEDLARS), which is a computerized literature retrieval service of the National Library of Medicine. That library's holdings exceed two and a half million books, journals, technical reports, theses, and other materials. A terminal computer in an on-line center that offers the MEDLARS service (usually a library in a school of medicine) is connected to the computer at the National Library of Medicine. To retrieve references, the computer carries on a dialogue with the user. The computer refines the search by asking and receiving answers to successive queries until the references are identified. The search takes 10 to 15 minutes, using subject headings or words that may appear in titles or abstracts. The computer can conduct in a short time a search that would take hours if done manually.

A computer printout of the retrieved references provides lists of the subject headings and abstracts. The printout can be simplified to include only elements necessary for retrieving the item, such as author, title, and source. Materials the user cannot locate elsewhere can be borrowed directly through the National Library of Medicine.

Anyone can have access to the MEDLARS search. The librarian will conduct the search or the user may be instructed how to do it. Fees for MEDLARS searches vary. Some of the regional centers with this capability do not charge at all; others may assess a minimal fee. Occasionally the search results will not be printed at the terminal but will be at the National Library of Medicine computer and mailed to the user.

## Textbooks and Journals

Textbooks are useful resources for use in continuing education. A review copy often will be sent by the publisher upon request. The publisher expects the text to be adopted so requests for review copies should be predicated upon anticipation that the book actually will be used in a continuing education class.

Many of the specialty nursing journals devote issues to a single subject that can constitute a valuable handout for participants. Publishers of these professional journals will send review copies for potential use in courses or workshops. There often are price discounts if the journal material is accepted for use. Many publishers grant subscription discounts to course participants. Care must be taken, however, so that it does not appear that the program is promoting a particular journal.

Voluntary health agencies have materials available for use in continuing education. Organizations such as the American Heart Association, Mental Health Association, American Red Cross, and others are excellent sources, as are professional associations. Many of these materials are available free or for a nominal charge.

Articles from professional journals are valuable resources. However, care must be taken not to violate the copyright laws. The program staff must be aware of these laws and the ethical and legal responsibility to comply. Photocopying articles from journals is covered by the copyright law that took effect January 1, 1980. Before reprinting articles for distribution, it is wise to seek permission from the publisher or author. The letter seeking permission to reprint copyrighted material should state specifically who the requester is, the institution represented, what articles or pages are sought, and what will be done with the reprints. Users must be sure to get the permission in writing.

Once permission is obtained, users must be careful to do only what was described—and no more. If the user finds the number of reprinted copies requested has been underestimated, the copyright holder must be so informed. Specific information about copyright laws and how they affect users can be obtained from any librarian. If a user has access to the library in a health-related college or university, it may already have established policies and procedures related to copyrighted material.

## Targeting the Resources

In selecting materials, it is useful to categorize them by their focus. For example, books, bibliographies, copies of journal articles, or audiotapes encourage abstract thinking or concept formation. Some resources such as films, demonstrations, and videotapes provide a learning experience through observation. Some allow participation in a simulated setting, such as a return-demonstration component where the instructor demonstrates and the participants return the demonstration to show mastery of the skill, role playing, simulation games, or case studies. Finally, there are resources that permit active participation in the real setting in which the learning is to be applied. The most common of these is clinical experience on a nursing unit, but some group discussions can be structured to allow for such an application to a real setting also.

Evaluation of the selected material resources is as important as it is of the human resources. Participants and planning committee members, as well as the continuing education staff, should evaluate the effectiveness of the resources used in the course. A checklist can be designed for this purpose. It can be standardized for any of the courses that use such resources. Questions on such a standardized form could include those specific to the handout materials; how long it should take to read them; and how readable, interesting, or appropriate they were. A file then can be kept on such materials as is the file on potential faculty, so that the best resources are cataloged and on tap for future use.

## FINANCIAL RESOURCES

Financial resources for continuing education are available from a variety of sources.

If a continuing education department is lucky, it will receive direct funding from the parent organization so that it does not spend more time looking for financial stability than it does on its programming. Sources of such in-house funding differ, based on the institution in which the department is located.

In any case, the program staff should develop and use a funding strategy to make the maximum use of available financial resources. The steps in developing such a strategy are to:

1. define the exact sum necessary to conduct the program
2. identify existing sources of income such as the funds provided by the parent institution, and the purposes for which these funds are provided
3. ascertain alternate or additional sources of funds such as grants, gifts, or in-kind services
4. determine what must be done to obtain other funds
5. decide, in order of priority, which actions to undertake to obtain these funds, based, of course, on the resources available in terms of time and energy

Of primary consideration, also, are the contraints under which the program must operate within an institution that may influence the kinds and types of other funds that can be sought. Without an appropriate tax status, for example, institutions cannot receive foundation funds, which may preclude their obtaining money from that source.

Among the many sources of funding available to a continuing education program are contracts, consultations, sales or rental of educational materials, gifts, fees for services, and others. Funds also are available through grants from private foundations and governments.

## Contracts

Contracts can be signed with outside agencies to obtain financial support. The contract is based on the program's offering a specific service, such as providing education on alcoholism to all management personnel in a local industry. Contracts can provide continuing education for employees of hospitals, either for specific departments such as nursing or for the institution's entire staff if that is within the program's capability.

Contracts must be written agreements, with the terms spelled out as precisely as possible in advance. While some latitude is advisable in terms of the hours, number of persons to be educated, subject areas, location, and so on, both parties must understand the terms and conditions to avoid any later misunderstandings that could have deleterious effects. The program planner may initiate the contract or the request may be made by the client agency.

If the planner develops the contract there must be sufficient evidence that the program can produce what it promises. Previous successful classes or courses on the subject help provide a track record. The evidence also can include the fact that grant funds were obtained for classes in that subject from another source.

## Consultation

The program planner may contract to consult with other agencies in providing education. In this case, the agency itself conducts the course but relies on the continuing education staff to provide the expertise since the agency may lack that talent. If the program planner receives funds from consultations, a decision must be made as to their disposition. The institution may have policies on consultation or the planner may initiate the decision on whether to return all or a percentage of the consulting funds to the continuing education program.

## Sales or Rentals

Financial gains (resources) can result from sales or rentals of educational materials developed by the continuing education program. The materials usually are developed for a specific course or workshop and are so well received that there are requests for copies. While it is generous of the program to share them without cost, if the staff have to generate much of their own income, such sales or rentals are attractive revenue-producers. If the materials are duplicated for rental or sale, their availability should be advertised to increase public awareness of their existence. If the continuing education department lacks the capability to reproduce the materials, their sale to a commercial firm that can publish and disseminate them should be considered. The commercial firm would pay royalties to the department. Royalties are based on a flat figure per unit or on a percentage of the profit after the cost of duplicating, publicizing, and distributing the materials is deducted. The income may be minimal but should not be overlooked.

## Gifts

Gifts from groups or individuals are another source of income but seldom involve major sums. Gifts should be made directly to the continuing education program, if feasible. If not, they may be made to the parent institution and earmarked for the program.

## Fees for Services

Fees for services probably comprise the majority of the funds available to the department. These are the fees charged for registration in the workshops, courses, or classes sponsored by the program. While the registration fees should cover the basic costs of the activity itself, they generally do not generate enough income to cover the expenses of the entire program. Raising fees enough to cover all such costs may result in prohibitive charges that would reduce attendance severely.

## Other Income Sources

Employers often budget funds to reimburse nurses for their participation in continuing education activities. Money also may be available to the individual nurse who wishes to participate in a course on high risk infants from an organization such as the March of Dimes, which is particularly interested in improving the skills of nurses working with high risk infants.

Money also is available directly to the continuing education program from organizations such as the American Red Cross or the voluntary health agencies such as heart, epilepsy, or multiple sclerosis. Requests should be directed to the organization well in advance of the time for the event so that they can move through the appropriate channels in the granting organization.

Groups such as a state's emergency medical services commission or commission on the aged and aging may have discretionary funds to provide continuing education for nurses working with the specific population of citizens for which the group has responsibility. Groups that focus on the humanities and arts often can make small grants to educational endeavors; for example, a class or course on values or ethics may meet the criteria for a humanities award.

## In-Kind Services

Although not direct income, other financial resources such as in-kind services should not be overlooked. The accounting, bookkeeping, mailing, and general administrative support available without charge from the parent institution is a source of indirect financial aid for the program. In a university, for example, faculty members may be assigned a number of hours per year to teach continuing education classes as part of their workload, and since no fee is paid for their services, this results in a saving for the department. When continuing education activities are moved to locations away from the hospital, or when they are cosponsored with the outside host agency, the latter may assume responsibility for registration, which is a timesaver (and hence cost-saver) for the staff development program.

## Volunteers

The use of volunteers (or students on work-study programs if the continuing education department is in a university) often is overlooked as a financial resource. Volunteers should not be used in place of regular staff in the program but can be on reserve for times of peak demand such as when catalogs or brochures are mailed out. Work-study students with appropriate skills can assume some of the clerical responsibilities in the department. Not to be overlooked is the potential for providing internships for students in curricula with some relationship to the program's mission. The assumption here is that the program planner is sincerely interested in serving as a preceptor for the student. As a trade-off, the student assists the planner in performing some work, but free labor should not be the motivation behind seeking out such opportunities.

Funding sources should be chosen with care so that the integrity and quality of the program are not compromised. Whenever possible, the continuing education department should have its own budget so that its income does not automatically go into the institution's general fund. Having one's own budget requires accounting and bookkeeping functions that are not necessary if the money goes into the general fund, but it also provides much more flexibility for the program director in handling the department's funds. Some institutions may expect any funds in excess of those required for operating the program to be turned over to the general fund at the end of the fiscal year. Many program planners are comfortable with that arrangement since in years in which there is a deficit, the parent institution assumes the costs, without the program's having to generate income to cover the loss. The result is a system of balances for the continuing education program.

## GRANTS

When deciding whether to seek grant support for a project, the program director must determine that it will be in the best interest of the parent organization. The project will have an impact on the institution in terms of time commitment, space requirements, and indirect costs that may not be reimbursed by the granting agency. The program must avoid fractionalizing staff and resources or becoming dependent on grant support for general operational expenses. Continuing education projects should extend, rather than supplement, the program's activities. In seeking grant support, the program director may apply to a private foundation or agency or to the government.

## Foundation Grants

Private foundations often provide money for short-term educational programs. The general guideline to be followed is to plan continuing education activities first, then to seek funds, rather than to plan events based on what funds are available.

The planner first must identify the appropriate foundation to approach for funds. Foundations generally have specific areas in which they provide funds, so that an approach to the wrong one will be an exercise in futility. Even if a foundation does grant funds in certain areas, it may not be interested in this request, so much groundwork is necessary in order to obtain money. Some foundations may support only initiation of projects, not their implementation; some may fund planning but not operations; some may provide only seed money and expect the applicant institution to match the funds (generally with in-kind services); others may fund only innovative projects, so a careful search of what has been done in a field would precede a request. Most foundations have guidelines, including what kinds of grants they give and to what kinds of entities. Valuable information can be obtained from organizations' annual reports; most foundations make them available on request.

The continuing education program director makes the initial contact with the foundation in a brief letter that seeks to determine the organization's interest in a project proposal. The inquiry letter should describe the requesting agency, its director, why it thinks it can accomplish the project described, and why it thinks the foundation may be interested in funding the request. The proposal should be attached to the inquiry letter. It should be a brief and concise description of what is intended.

The proposal should describe the fundamental problem, subject, or issue as well as any corrective action (if appropriate). The project's objectives and specific contributions it is expected to make should be included. Since most of the reviewers of the proposal will not be familiar with the project's circumstances, it is essential that the details be spelled out, corrective measures identified (if a problem is involved), and the anticipated outcomes predicted as explicitly as possible. References to literature that support identification of the project (and possible solutions for a problem) should be included in a bibliography.

The proposal should be organized clearly and, if it is lengthy, should contain a table of contents. It is imperative to include a description of how the project will be evaluated. The proposed budget should cover the costs of all of the project's activities. All budget items should be related to those referred to in the proposal.

It should go without saying that a proposal or letter of inquiry that is poorly written or contains grammatical or spelling errors will have an adverse effect on the reviewer. Care should be taken in typing and reproducing copies of both the letter and the proposal.

The letter should state that the project director will call the foundation to check on its status in about two weeks after it has had time to review the proposal. The director then should follow through. The proposal should be sent to a specific individual in the foundation to avoid the consequences of a "Dear Sir" or a "To whom it may concern" letter.

When the foundation responds to the letter of inquiry and the brief project outline, the real work of preparing a proposal for funding begins. A favorable response from the staff of a private foundation often means that the proposal has an excellent chance of being funded. Staff members can pass on information that will facilitate the writing of the proposal and its subsequent funding. The project director should listen carefully and be prepared to implement the suggestions.

### Methods of Submission

Private foundations generally have two methods for the submission of proposals:

1. The material necessary to flesh out the proposal is submitted to the foundation staff as needed. The information should be complete and sent as promptly as possible. It is important to understand exactly what is being requested; because of the foundation's relative unfamiliarity with the proposal, its staff may have to seek clarification to be sure the appropriate materials are being sent. The foundation staff then write up the proposal (usually with a positive—or a negative—recommendation) and submit it to the appropriate group in the foundation for action.
2. The project director is responsible for submitting the proposal following the foundation's guidelines. In this case also, the foundation staff will be of invaluable assistance in preparing the proposal. The funding guidelines must be studied carefully so that the director understands what information is required. This will help avoid overlooking necessary information that would delay the processing of the application. If there are deadlines listed, they must be met. Ample time must be allowed to obtain approvals within the requesting or applicant agency before the final proposal is submitted to the foundation.

If certain information is to be placed in certain sections of the report according to the guidelines, the director must be sure to do so. Important information may be missed if the reviewer is looking in one section and the project director has placed it in another. Proposals that contain excess words, exaggerated claims, excessive justification, and overworked jargon are not likely to be well received by a funding agency.

After the proposal is written and submitted, all the continuing education department can do is wait for a response. It is not effective to follow up a submission with frequent phone calls and letters; the foundation will notify the director when it has acted on the proposal.

If the proposal is rejected, the foundation should be asked for specific reasons why. Most foundations will provide fairly specific information that can be used to improve the proposal before it is resubmitted. The foundation staff may be able to say whether the proposal stands a chance if it is revised and resubmitted. Again, the project director must listen carefully and follow the specific instructions. If the foundation's funding guidelines have been followed properly, however, a rewrite and resubmission should not be necessary.

*The Project Review Process*

Project review varies by foundation, but there are several steps through which each proposal goes during the process. The reviewers ask questions such as these:

1. Does the proposal fit into the funding pattern of the foundation? If it does not, it will not be reviewed further. For that reason it is essential to be certain before submission that it is being sent to the appropriate foundation.
2. Does the proposal duplicate any other foundation program, past or present? Again, the need for research into the foundation's funding activities is obvious. Some foundations use experts in various fields as program consultants to apprise them of duplications. Their staffs also have contact with those of others and so can check on duplication among as well as within foundations. In the event that a project duplicates another that is being considered, the reviewers' response to the next several steps may determine which of the proposals receives funding, although the submission date may be the deciding factor.
3. Does the proposal address an issue or problem of significance? This is the step at which the clarity and preparation of the proposal are paramount. If the project director was luckless enough to seek funds from the wrong foundation, for the wrong program, or at the wrong time, there is little that can be salvaged by a good proposal. By this point,

however, all these considerations have been handled; it now is the proposal itself that is being judged. Documentation from others than the proposal writer may be helpful in establishing the significance of the project. Care should be taken that letters of support that accompany a proposal do not look like carbon copies of each other. If the proposal describes a project that has never been attempted, the reviewer has nothing to compare the possible results to, so the important aspects of the project, its outcomes, and its ramifications must be conceptualized accurately and stated precisely.

4. Does the proposal state possible outcomes? Here the reviewer looks not only at the outcomes the writer has specified but also at possible spinoffs from the proposal. In addition, the reviewer carefully considers whether this project may serve as a model for others.

5. Does the proposal specify how much it will cost? At this point, and generally only now, is the expense of the project reviewed. The question to be answered here is whether the project is worth what it will cost. If the director has carefully built a case for the significance and possible outcomes of the project and if the budget seems in line, this step will be simple. Foundation staff experts are quick to note padded budget estimates, so budgets must be kept simple and in line. The budget items should be justified where appropriate, such as when equipment is to be purchased.

6. Does the department submitting the proposal seem able to carry it out effectively? The foundation at this point reviews the qualifications of the project managers. If they already are on staff, their vitae submitted with the proposal should be current and should reflect their ability to handle an operation of these dimensions. Foundation staff may respond to this step or any of the others through personal interviews with the individuals making the funding request. Staff members from the foundation may visit the requesting agency or may invite individuals to visit them. In the event that foundation staff visit the department, it is essential that all of the individuals who were required to sign the proposal application are knowledgeable about the project and supportive of it.

Upon receiving satisfactory responses to these questions, the foundation staff can then present the proposal to its funding body for approval. Funding bodies in foundations vary. Staff members usually have the responsibility for initial screening of proposals and presentation to the approval body, often with recommendations to accept or reject. Staff members serve as liaison between the approval body and the fund requesters.

Foundations usually have express requirements on publicity and acknowledgment of the grant support they have provided. In addition to following these requirements, the department director should be generous with ac-knowledgments of the support, including sending the foundation newsclip-pings referring to the project. The director must be sure to separate recognition for the foundation from that of corporations that may have the same name.

The prudent project director reports progress to the foundation on at least an annual basis; most foundations require such reporting while others do not, but it's a good idea to keep in touch.

## Federal Grants

Grant funds also are available from the federal government for continuing education activities. The initial step is to obtain the guidelines for writing the proposal. Those guidelines must be followed to the letter. The proposal is competing for money as well as for the reviewers' time, so it is essential that the format be followed meticulously.

The basic information needed in a proposal submitted for federal funding includes these elements:

1. A title page should include the name of the applicant, the applicant's agency name, dates of the project, total budget request, and signatures of those in the agency required to approve such proposals.
2. An abstract should summarize the project's purpose, objectives, evaluation, and dissemination. The abstract should not be longer than two pages, preferably much shorter.
3. A statement of the problem should be documented by a review of the related literature, if appropriate. This statement should include the effects if the issue is not addressed. Reference can be made to previous projects that attest to the need for this one, if applicable. This section should make the significance of the project clear to the reviewer.
4. The project's objectives should be stated clearly and should be measurable. There should be one objective for each area identified in the section on the statement of the problem. The objectives should be realistic for the time allotted.
5. The procedures through which the objectives will be met should be described in an overall approach, followed by specific activities designed to achieve them. Included in this section are the population to be served, the administration and management of the project, and the time needed to accomplish the objectives. There should be a description for each objective.
6. The evaluation of the attainment of the objectives should state explicitly the type of evaluative information to be collected, how it will be analyzed, and how it will be used.

7. The dissemination of information about the project should be described, including how it will be shared with others and how the funding agency will be kept apprised of the activities.
8. The next information needed is a description of the facilities that will house the project. This section should describe all of the support services, such as computers, libraries, and so on that will contribute to the project.
9. The individuals who will be responsible for the project should be described, including those already employed and those who will be needed. The expertise of those already employed to manage a project of this kind should be evident.
10. The final step of the project proposal should be a detailed budget. This should include the categories of personnel (salaries and fringe benefits), equipment, travel, supplies, and expenses. Indirect costs charged by the parent agency for a project vary with the institution; the latest figures should be checked and included, along with the value of in-kind services provided by the host agency.

When the proposal has been completed, it should answer the questions:

- Why does it need to be done? (Section on statement of the problem.)

- What will be done? (Section on objectives.)

- How will it be done? (Sections on procedures, evaluation, and dissemination.)

- Who will be involved? (Sections on facilities and personnel.)

- How much will it cost? (Section on budget.)

Materials to clarify or expand the proposal should be provided in the appendixes. These may include an additional description of the geographic area in which the project will take place, the institution in which it will be housed, demographic data on the population to be served, and letters of support from key individuals and groups. Only materials that contribute to the substance of the proposal should be in the appendixes; there should be no materials included just for filler.

Specific deadlines for federal projects should be adhered to closely. A panel of reviewers selects proposals that meet the criteria for funding. The situation is most competitive, so that it is essential that the proposal meet all the criteria and be written in a manner that does not deviate from the guidelines for federal funding.

## GRANTS WRITING

The continuing education director can become skilled at obtaining outside funding for projects related to the department's activities. Essential to success at grants writing is knowing the basic needs and problems in the parent institution housing the program. These basic needs must be expressed clearly and concisely in any proposal. The needs also must be substantiated, preferably by hard data, to which the program has access through its research and evaluation activities.

Knowledge of funding sources is important so that an agency making grants in the appropriate area can be contacted. Time should not be wasted in submitting grant proposals to the wrong agency.

The director also can work to establish the institution's commitment to projects by involving key persons in the organization in the program. Evidence of successful interrelationships and support within an organization for a project will strengthen any project proposal.

The program director must develop access to information about funding sources, such as a library that has the literature from various agencies, as well as current bulletins and application forms. A person in the department who is a grants writer to whom the director can turn for assistance is an invaluable resource. If not, the continuing education director may choose to be the person who keeps up with funding programs, guidelines, and deadlines for other departments in the institution. Getting on the mailing list of funding agencies will ensure that the most up-to-date information is received in timely fashion.

Grant funds from private foundations and the federal government can increase the visibility of the continuing education department and enhance its standing in the institution. The effort to seek outside sources of income quite often has payoffs beyond those associated merely with the receipt of the funds.

---

**SUGGESTED READINGS**

Brown, M. Alan, and Copeland, Harlan G., eds. *Attracting Able Instructors of Adults:* 4 (San Francisco: Jossey-Bass, Inc.), 1979.

Lewis, Marianna, ed. *The Foundation Directory,* 6th ed. New York: Russell Sage Foundation, 1977.

*The Foundation Center National Data Book.* New York: The Foundation Center, 1977.

U.S. Department of Health, Education, and Welfare. *NIH Guide for Grants and Contracts.* Washington, D.C.: U.S. Government Printing Office, 1972.

U.S. Office of Management and Budget. *Catalog of Federal Domestic Assistance.* Washington, D.C.: U.S. Government Printing Office, 1975.

# Chapter 8

# The Action Plan and Implementation

The responsibility for detailed planning usually falls to the staff of continuing education in nursing or other designated persons in the institution. This phase of the development of a continuing education course is crucial to its success. No matter how well a planning committee has outlined the needs, objectives, content, and methods for presenting subject matter and has assisted in identifying the potential resources, the activity will not succeed unless the staff assume responsibility for moving from the generalized to detailed planning.

## BUDGET

The budget, which has been discussed, also is considered a part of resource identification. A general outline of the budget should be included in the early work of the planning committee. However, at this later phase of development it is necessary to formalize the budget as a part of the detailed planning. The appropriate budget forms should be prepared and approval obtained from the appropriate persons in the institution. Policies should be established that indicate what budgeting approvals are necessary. For example, if a university is the sponsor and has a separate continuing education department, the budget may have to be approved only by the director of that department; in a hospital, it may have to be processed through the director of nursing to the administrator.

## FACULTY

One of the first steps in the detailed planning is contacting potential faculty members for the continuing education activity. The planning committee already has made a number of suggestions and set priorities for the persons it would like to have conduct the course. The initial contact can be by telephone or letter. The faculty member should be informed of the objectives, the desired general content, the number of persons expected to attend, dates, place, time allotted, and any other faculty instructors the program director would like to participate or intends to contact. The instructor should be informed of the instructional fee and travel expenses. It is helpful to have a faculty salary scale based on educational qualifications and experience. This can be established on a per hour or per day basis. The per hour basis provides more flexibility, since instructors may teach only a part of a session and it is easier to figure payment on an hourly basis.

A salary scale makes it easier to plan for instructional costs and allows for some flexibility in payments. It also is a fairer system since the program does not find itself paying different amounts to persons with equal qualifications. Of course, there will be situations where experts will have a set fee and are not willing to vary from it. The planning committee needs to be aware of this fact and, if it is seeking that type of resource person, check out the fee at the early stage. Faculty travel expenses are budgeted under the institution's guidelines. Most organizations have a per mile fee for automobile travel and per diem for meals and motel or hotel expenses. The instructor should be made aware of what the institution will reimburse for expenses.

If the faculty member agrees to teach the continuing education course or class, follow-up contact should be made in writing. The letter should include a copy of the planning committee's minutes on this course and the objectives, content, and suggested teaching methods and resource materials. It should be understood that there is room for negotiation and the instructor has the freedom to alter the committee's suggestions.

At this time it is important to obtain a written agreement with the faculty member. The agreement should include the name of the continuing education activity, the date, time, hours, location, maximum enrollment, minimum enrollment required to conduct the course, and payment of the teacher for instruction and expenses. An example of the agreement is shown in Exhibit 8-1. This agreement assures an understanding of expectations between the faculty member and the institution and alleviates misunderstandings about fee payments, dates, or hours. Two copies are sent to the faculty member, one to be signed and returned and the other to be retained by the teacher.

In this communication with the faculty it is important to set a time period for follow-up to discuss any changes in objectives, content, teaching methods,

**Exhibit 8-1** Example of a Faculty Agreement

---

MEMORANDUM OF TEMPORARY OR PART-TIME APPOINTMENT

NAME: _____

ADDRESS: _____

TELEPHONE: Office _____ Home _____ Social Security _____

ACTIVITY TITLE: _____

LOCATION: _____

DATE(S): _____ MINIMUM ENROLLMENT: _____

OMIT DATE(S): _____ MAXIMUM ENROLLMENT: _____

DAY(S) OF WEEK: _____ COMPENSATION

TIME: _____ INSTRUCTION: _____

TRAVEL: _____

OTHER: _____

THE FOLLOWING NOTES AND CONDITIONS ARE PART OF YOUR APPOINTMENT:

1. If the minimum number of enrollments indicated above does not materialize, the program may not be offered and the University will have no financial obligation to you.

2. In the event that it is impossible for you to instruct the entire course, your compensation will be adjusted according to specific costs and expenses incurred by us in finding a replacement, rescheduling or canceling the program, and refunding the fees.

3. It is assumed by your signature on this appointment that you have received approval from your institution or organization to teach this course.

Instructor's Signature _____ Date _____

Program Coordinator's Signature _____ Date _____

Revised 6/18/79

*Source:* Reprinted with permission from the *Departmental Operating Manual,* Division of Continuing Studies, Columbus Campus, Indiana University-Purdue University at Indianapolis, ©1979.

and so on. If possible, the director should arrange to meet with the teacher to wrap up details of the workshop. However, this frequently is unrealistic in terms of time involved in travel and the location of the individual. Ideally, the faculty person should meet with the planning committee, but again this may not be easy to arrange because of time and expense.

## MATERIALS AND AUDIOVISUALS

To initiate other phases of detailed planning, it is advisable to discuss with the faculty member the audiovisual materials, books, and/or resource materials suggested by the planning committee. The instructor may suggest additional materials. The audiovisual equipment required may influence the decision on the location of the workshop or course. If books are required, these must be ordered well in advance, and films must be reserved. It is essential that this information be included in the budget and fee structure. Materials the instructor may wish to have duplicated for participants should be clarified and the time frame for receiving them for preparation established. The teacher should supply an up-to-date vita and any additional information needed for processing the forms for payment.

Unless the department has its own audiovisual equipment, it must be reserved through the appropriate other department. The university or hospital may have an audiovisual department that not only will supply the equipment but also will arrange for setting it up for the course. This relieves the program coordinator of a major responsibility. However, if this service is not available, the director should be sure to know how to run the equipment or where to acquire an operator.

The agency should have policies related to the use of audiovisual equipment. Reserving the equipment early in the planning process assures the director that it will be available on the day(s) needed. In reserving the equipment the program director must check to make sure there is an ample supply of extra bulbs on hand and, if the workshop is outside the facility, that an extra bulb accompanies each machine. Audiovisual materials are a great adjunct to a presentation but only when the equipment functions well.

Planners must request audiovisual software if it is not being provided by the instructor. The planning committee may have identified a particular 16mm film that can be used to present one segment of the content. The instructor concurs with the use of the film. Before including this in the schedule, the director must determine where the film can be obtained free or on a rental basis (and the cost) and whether it will be available on the date needed. A written confirmation should be obtained before it is included in the budget. The instructor who plans to use slides, tapes, or transparencies usually provides these. Filmstrips or audiotapes may be rented from an outside source. As with a 16mm film, it is essential to locate a source, determine the cost, and obtain a written confirmation before listing them on the schedule.

## FACILITY

The choice of location should be based on the type of activity and the accommodations needed. If the course is planned for one or two days or a series of short sessions over a period of weeks, the site could be the university or hospital, a local facility that is available free, or a motel or hotel at reasonable terms. A facility checklist (Exhibit 8-2) may be used as a guide in surveying a location to determine its usability.

The use of space in your own facility usually is the simplest for staff in terms of making arrangements and conducting a course. The staff are familiar with the space, room setups for groups of various sizes, audiovisual equipment, and other services available. Although this may be the most convenient for the staff, the facility's accessibility and parking may be a problem for participants, and these factors should be considered. There may be a problem scheduling space in a college, university, or hospital, so the use of other facilities may be necessary.

Planning committee members may have suggestions for community facilities that are available free or at low cost. Shopping centers may have conference rooms or auditoriums that are reasonable in price and provide the type of room setup required for an educational workshop. Vocational schools, churches, and local business firms are other potential facilities that may have space available, are accessible to participants, and are willing to accommodate nursing courses.

If a more intensive educational workshop is planned that will be held over a period of days or weeks, overnight accommodations for participants, faculty, and staff as well as facilities for conducting the course will be needed. The design of the activity may require a "retreat" atmosphere where participants, faculty, and staff will be able to concentrate in a casual, uninterrupted atmosphere. Arrangements for this type of facility must be made well in advance since demand for their use usually is high.

In arranging for a location that includes overnight accommodations, it will be necessary to provide information about the approximate number of persons, the numbers and types (singles, doubles) of rooms to be held (and their prices), as well as the meeting rooms (and their cost). A decision must be made on whether the sponsor or the participants will make the reservations. If participants are to make their reservations, then appropriate cards should be included in the advance information kits. Agreement should be reached with the facility on the date for a final guarantee for the reserved rooms. It

**Exhibit 8-2** Sample of List for Surveying a Location

```
                            FACILITY CHECKLIST

Name of Activity:
Location:
Contact Person:
Telephone Number:


I.    Space
      A.  Size of room adequate for        Classroom style _____ Number _____
          number of persons and           Theater style   _____ Number _____
          teaching strategy

      B.  Breakout rooms for small         # of rooms available ____ size _____
          group sessions                  NA _____

      C.  Chairs designed for comfort      Yes _____ No _____
          of adults

      D.  Various sizes and shapes of      Yes _____ No _____ NA _____
          tables available                Describe:


      E.  Audiovisual equipment available  Yes _____ No _____ NA _____
                                           Additional fee for use: (amount) _____
                                           Type(s) available:


      F.  Cost for rental of space is      Yes _____ No _____ Amount _____
          reasonable

      G.  Lighting                         Good ____ Adequate ____ Poor ____

      H.  Acoustics                        Good ____ Adequate ____ Poor ____

      I.  Extraneous noises                Minimal ____ Acceptable level ____

      J.  Ventilation                      Good ____ Adequate ____ Poor ____

      K.  Temperature control              Good ____ Adequate ____ Poor ____


II.   Participant Accomodations
      A.  Overnight rooms available        Yes _____ No _____ NA _____

      B.  Food service available on:
          1.  a planned menu basis         Yes _____ No _____ NA _____
          2.  individual selection         Yes _____ No _____ NA _____

      C.  Refreshment service available    Yes _____ No _____ NA _____

      D.  Adequate restroom facilities     Yes _____ No _____ NA _____
          available for number of
          participants
```

**Exhibit 8-2** continued

III.  Accessibility

    A.  Location easily accessible by        Yes _____  No _____
        automobile

    B.  Location easily accessible by        Yes _____  No _____  NA _____
        public transportation

    C.  Adequate parking with adequate       Yes _____  No _____  NA _____
        security

Other comments:

*Source:* Reprinted with permission from the *Departmental Operating Manual*, Division of Continuing Studies, Columbus Campus, Indiana University-Purdue University at Indianapolis, ©1980.

is important to ascertain the checkout hour and make arrangements for participants if the event extends beyond that time on the last day.

Written agreements should be made with the facility. If the course is being conducted in your own facility, a room reservation form (Exhibit 8-3) may be all that is necessary. This form can be used as a guide in establishing a system for reserving space if you do not have one. It also serves as a guide in formalizing an agreement for use of space in any facility.

For any space arrangements, there must be an understanding about the desired conference room arrangement, the number of persons expected, and the type of equipment (and whether the sponsor or the facility is providing it). A drawing of the precise layout (Exhibit 8-4) eliminates disagreements. The continuing education program may be bringing its own audiovisual equipment but need a cart or table for this equipment and an extension cord with a three-way socket. The registration setup and its location, as well as space for display materials, must be arranged. All of this should be specified in writing when reserving space. A clear advance understanding between the sponsor and the facility serves to avoid confusion on the day of the workshop.

## MEALS AND REFRESHMENTS

A decision must be made about meals for workshop participants. If the event is being held in a motel or hotel, it usually is necessary to eat there to avoid a charge for the meeting room. The requirements for a meal or meals as part of the agreement to use the facility should be clarified in the initial contact. The menu should be reviewed to determine meal options and prices. It should be realized that whatever food is chosen will not please everyone.

**Exhibit 8-3** Sample Conference Reservation Form

```
              ROOM RESERVATION FORM               MUST BE SUBMITTED TWO
                                                  WEEKS IN ADVANCE
            COLUMBUS CAMPUS OF IUPUI              Check One:
                 2080 Bakalar Drive               ☐ New Request
              Columbus, Indiana 47201             ☐ Change of Earlier Request
                                                  ☐ Cancellation of Request
```

Item
No.

1. Name of Organization_____

2. Person Making Request_____
                                (Name)              (Bus. Phone)   (Home Phone)

   _____

3. Room(s) Requested_____Date of Request_____

4. Date(s) of Event_____

5. Hour(s) of Meeting   From_____AM   _____PM    ROOM MUST BE SET-UP BY:
                        To_____AM     _____PM    DATE_____ TIME_____

6. Name & Type of
   Program or Activity_____

   _____

            Will admission fee be charged?   YES____    NO____

7. Expected Attendance_____

8. Special Equipment Needed:

   Furniture (Specify Quantity):
                              Classroom
      Folding Chairs_____    Arm Chairs_____   Tables (Round)_____   Tables (Other)_____

      Ash Trays_____   Speaker's Podium_____   Speaker's Platform_____

   Audio Visual:

      Tape Recorder_____   Portable Screen_____   Movie Projector_____   TV Monitor_____

      Overhead Projector_____   Slide Projector_____   Record Player_____

      Other_____

9. Special Seating Arrangements:   YES_____   NO_____   (Attach diagram if YES)

10. Miscellaneous_____

11. Special Personnel Needed  (Involves Overtime Pay Beyond Regular Hours):

    Custodial_____Physical Plant_____ Other (Specify)_____

------------------------------------------------------------------------------

                  (FOR BUSINESS OFFICE USE ONLY)

12. Room(s) Assigned_____Confirmation Sent_____By_____

13. Room Usage Fee_____Estimated Charge For Personnel (See Line 11)_____


    DISTRIBUTION:

    (1)  Business Office   (2)  Calendar Office   (3)   Building Services  (4)  Applicant

*Source:* Reprinted with permission from the *Departmental Operating Manual,* Division of Continuing Studies, Columbus Campus, Indiana University-Purdue University at Indianapolis, ©1980.

**Exhibit 8-4** Sample Conference Room Layouts

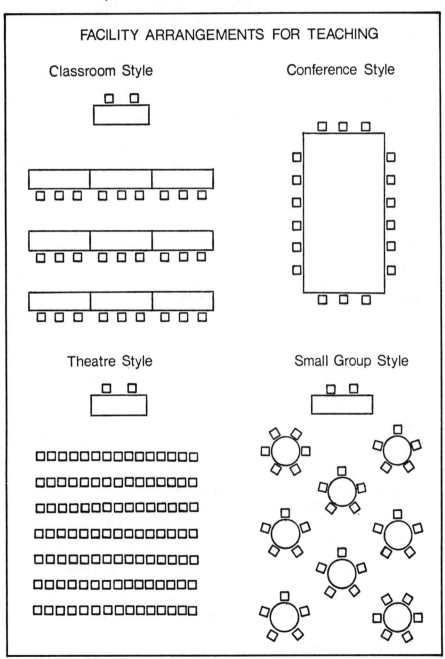

The meal cost may be so unrealistic that it will be decided not to use the facility. It is important to know the deadline for giving a final count for meals and what leeway is possible in terms of last-minute cancellations.

If the workshop location is not convenient to eating facilities, it may be necessary to have the meals catered. The facility should be able to provide a list of caterers used previously or the program planners may know caterers in the area. The caterer should be given a price range that the conference can afford and determine what can be served within that cost. It must be remembered that the price of meals must be passed on to the participants and will increase the cost of the event for them as well as for the sponsor since the cost for the instructors' meals must be included.

If the meal is not a part of the workshop cost and the nurses are on their own, a list of nearby restaurants must be included in the packet of materials. If the conference is held in a health care institution and participants will eat in the cafeteria, the dietitian or food service manager must be informed of the number of extra persons to serve. (The dietitian also might be concerned about outsiders' impressions about the food and prefer to make some alteration in the menu.)

Another very important arrangement is for coffee at registration and at breaks. It is necessary to check on the cost of coffee per person, whether hot tea also can be made available, and whether soft drinks can be available during the afternoon break (and at what prices). If the workshop is being conducted in-house, these arrangements must be made with the appropriate persons there.

Meals and coffee are very important to the physical and psychological environment for the activity. Nurses participating in continuing education courses have come to expect that these needs will be taken care of and may express frustration if they find no coffee or tea available. Many good discussions and exchanges of ideas and experiences occur over a cup of coffee or while eating lunch together. Comments to this effect frequently are found on the "satisfaction or happiness index" completed at the end of the event.

Transportation and housing for out-of-town faculty must be arranged. Motel or hotel reservations should be made well in advance, with confirmation sent directly to the faculty person. Most hotels or motels will hold the reservation for late arrival on a guarantee from the sponsor. Travel arrangements may include making plane reservations and providing transportation from the airport. It is essential to clarify whether the program planners or faculty members are making these arrangements, since the latter may want to handle their own travel arrangements. Travel costs must be clarified to determine whether payment will be in advance or on a reimbursement basis. This should be included in the faculty agreement and the necessary forms processed if an advance payment is required.

## MARKETING THE EVENT

How is the continuing education in nursing event to be advertised or marketed? This decision must be made early in the planning process. There are budgeting implications for the method chosen. The type of announcement to be used and the information to be included, how it will be circulated, and to whom, are decisions to be made by the planning committee and the staff. If the decision requires design, printing/duplicating, and mailing of information in some form such as a brochure, the staff will have to make the arrangements. The lead time required by the print shop must be determined and the mailing list compiled or requested if the information is to be mailed. (For more detailed information on marketing, see Chapter 3.)

## OTHER STAFF RESPONSIBILITIES

The staff person responsible for continuing education and the department secretary are primarily responsible for the detailed planning for the workshops or courses. Since they may be working on several activities at the same time, a checklist is essential to determine whether all details are being handled and what phase of planning has been reached for each event on a day-by-day basis. The checklist should denote each step of the planning, implementation, and follow-up process in sequence and detail the responsibilities of both the staff person and the secretary in sequence. In establishing responsibilities, some duplication may be found and eliminated. It may be difficult to remember every detail in developing the first checklist, so frequent revisions may be necessary. However, once the checklists are set, they are invaluable in ensuring that all arrangements are being handled (Exhibits 8-5 and 8-6). Each organization will have different requirements based on its policies and procedures. For example, payment forms and procedures differ. Universities may have several methods for paying continuing education faculty members, depending on such factors as their full-time employment status (university or nonuniversity) and the length of time the individuals will teach. The staff person is responsible for determining the type of payment form and informing the secretary. In staff development of a health care facility, the procedure may be less complicated.

## FINAL PLANNING

Once the minimum number of registrations has been received, the final planning begins. The first step is to prepare for duplication of materials. If the instructors have not submitted materials for duplication, they should be reminded (or prodded) as to the absolute deadline for reproduction. The staff

**Exhibit 8-5** Example of Checklist for Staff Organizer

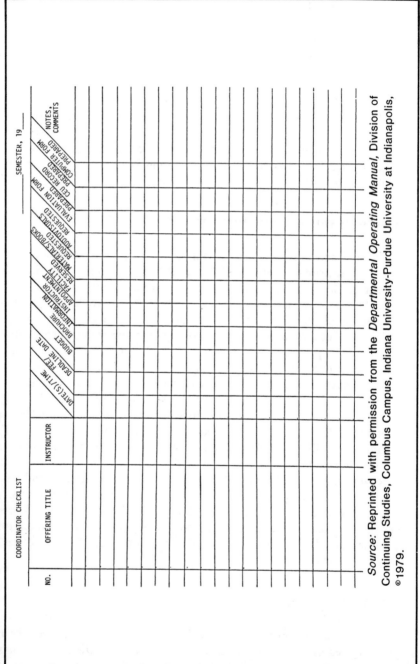

*Source:* Reprinted with permission from the *Departmental Operating Manual*, Division of Continuing Studies, Columbus Campus, Indiana University-Purdue University at Indianapolis, ©1979.

**Exhibit 8-6** Example of Checklist for Staff Secretary

```
                    SECRETARY - COURSE CHECKLIST

TITLE _____  NO. _____

DATES _____  LIMIT _____

INSTRUCTOR _____  LOCATION _____
```

ACTIVITY BUDGET

_____ Typed

_____ Signed and Approved

_____ Distributed

INSTRUCTOR(S)

Memorandum of Appointment:

_____ Sent

_____ Returned

Employee's Witholding Form (W-4):

_____ Sent

_____ Returned

Personal History:

_____ Sent

_____ Returned

   VITA   (New Appointments only):

_____ Sent

_____ Returned

Affirmative Action (New Appointments only):

_____ Sent

_____ Returned

ROOM REQUEST (to Business Office/Other Facility)

_____ Sent

_____ Confirmed, Room Number _____

BROCHURE

_____ Layout Completed

_____ Sent to Print Shop

_____ Returned from Print Shop

_____ Labels Requested

_____ Labels Received

_____ Mailed

SUPPLIES

_____ Requested

_____ Received

List:

PROMOTION

_____ News Release Written

_____ Mailed

TEXTBOOKS

_____ Ordered:

   Bookstore ☐

   Publisher ☐

_____ Received

AUDIOVISUAL EQUIPMENT

_____ Reserved

Type of Equipment:

Revised 5/80

**Exhibit 8-6** continued

INSTRUCTOR(S)　A. _____　　D. _____
　　　　　　　　　B. _____　　E. _____
　　　　　　　　　C. _____　　F. _____

| | | A | B | C | D | E | F |
|---|---|---|---|---|---|---|---|
| 1. | Payroll forms prepared | | | | | | |
| 2. | Payroll forms signed | | | | | | |
| 3. | Travel request prepared | | | | | | |
| 4. | Travel request signed | | | | | | |
| 5. | Travel voucher prepared | | | | | | |
| 6. | Travel voucher signed | | | | | | |
| 7. | Copies filed | | | | | | |
| 8. | Checks mailed | | | | | | |

MATERIALS TO PRINTER

_____ Handouts received
_____ To Printshop
_____ Printed
_____ Ready for class
_____ Evaluation to Printshop
_____ Printed
_____ CEU to Printshop
_____ Printed
_____ Agenda to Printshop
_____ Printed

REFRESHMENTS, MEALS

Supplies:

_____ Cups
_____ Coffee/Tea
_____ Sugar/Cream
_____ Napkins/Spoons
　　　　 Other (List):

Lunches:

_____ Initial Contact
　　　　 Person _____
_____ Requisition with Brochure
_____ Confirm Lunch Order
　　　　 Time: _____ No. _____

FIRST CLASS (check off)

_____ Roster
_____ Folders
_____ Room signs prepared
_____ Room signs posted
_____ Name tags/badges
_____ Computer forms
_____ Instruction sheets
_____ Evaluation
_____ Handouts

LAST CLASS (check off)

_____ Participant Certificates
　　　　 or CEU Record Prepared
_____ Student Evaluations

AFTER LAST CLASS (check off)

_____ Computer forms mailed
_____ Absentee Mailings
_____ Evaluations summarized
　　　　 Copy of Evaluation to:
　　　　 Instructor
　　　　 for nursing, B. Puetz
　　　　 Assistant Director of C.E.

CANCELLATION

_____ Course Cancellation Memo sent
_____ Instructor notified
_____ Enrollees notified
　　　　 (telephone/memo)
_____ Request for Return of
　　　　 Registration Fees processed

*Source:* Reprinted with permission from the *Departmental Operating Manual,* Division of Continuing Studies, Columbus Campus, Indiana University-Purdue University at Indianapolis, ©1980.

coordinator reviews the materials with the secretary and establishes the number of copies needed. It is helpful to have the materials duplicated on different colors of paper to help instructors and participants easily identify a particular handout being discussed and to number handout material and put it in the folder in the order of use.

If certificates or continuing education unit (CEU) records are being given for the course, these need to be prepared for duplication; if a CEU record, the course information should be included before reproduction.

Other forms may need to be prepared and duplicated for insertion in the packet, such as computer registration blanks containing course information and brochures outlining the schedule. A schedule for the session containing the objectives, faculty, schedule, and any other pertinent information must be prepared and duplicated, including an evaluation tool for each participant to provide written feedback.

Once all materials are duplicated, the coordinator reviews with the secretary how they are to be organized for distribution. A packet also should be prepared for each faculty member and the coordinator.

The preparation and use of nametags or namecards must be decided and the secretary instructed on how to prepare them. For example, if the workshop lasts only one day, stick-on tags may be fine; however, if it runs for several days, a more durable tag is needed. If participants will be seated around a table, namecards may be preferable; they can be used over a longer period and make it easier for the faculty to learn the names of the participants since they are easier to read from a distance.

A folder of materials must be prepared for the coordinator containing the roster of participants (Exhibit 8-7); extra nametags or cards, registration forms, payroll and travel forms that require the signatures of faculty members, and vita sheets for introducing faculty. The extra nametags or namecards and registration forms are necessary for persons who may arrive without having preregistered or if there are last-minute substitutions.

A last-minute check on equipment and audiovisual materials is imperative. The final number of meals should be given to the facility or caterers if meals are included. Purchase requisitions for meals, coffee, or rentals must be prepared if not done earlier. This is a good time to review both the coordinator and secretary checklists to make sure all details have been handled.

Workshops or courses conducted away from the health care institution or university involve being sure that all materials and equipment are ready and packed. The coordinator and secretary should be involved in this process.

Materials for distribution to participants at registration time should be checked and packed in a separate box and labeled. If additional materials are to be distributed, these are packaged and labeled separately as to the time they are to be handed out.

**Exhibit 8-7** Example of Roster of Participants / Attendance Checklist

CLASS ROSTER

OFFERING TITLE: _____ OFFERING # _____

CONDUCTED FOR: _____

DATES/TIME: _____

LOCATION: _____

INSTRUCTOR(S): _____

COORDINATOR: _____

| PARTICIPANTS (Last name, first name) | RN LPN OTHER | 1 | 2 | 3 | 4 | 5 | 6 | 7 | 8 | 9 | 10 | 11 | 12 |
|---|---|---|---|---|---|---|---|---|---|---|---|---|---|
| 1. | | | | | | | | | | | | | |
| 2. | | | | | | | | | | | | | |
| 3. | | | | | | | | | | | | | |
| 4. | | | | | | | | | | | | | |
| 5. | | | | | | | | | | | | | |
| 6. | | | | | | | | | | | | | |
| 7. | | | | | | | | | | | | | |
| 8. | | | | | | | | | | | | | |
| 9. | | | | | | | | | | | | | |
| 10. | | | | | | | | | | | | | |
| 11. | | | | | | | | | | | | | |
| 12. | | | | | | | | | | | | | |
| 13. | | | | | | | | | | | | | |
| 14. | | | | | | | | | | | | | |
| 15. | | | | | | | | | | | | | |
| 16. | | | | | | | | | | | | | |
| 17. | | | | | | | | | | | | | |
| 18. | | | | | | | | | | | | | |
| 19. | | | | | | | | | | | | | |
| 20. | | | | | | | | | | | | | |
| 21. | | | | | | | | | | | | | |
| 22. | | | | | | | | | | | | | |
| 23. | | | | | | | | | | | | | |
| 24. | | | | | | | | | | | | | |
| 25. | | | | | | | | | | | | | |
| 26. | | | | | | | | | | | | | |
| 27. | | | | | | | | | | | | | |
| 28. | | | | | | | | | | | | | |
| 29. | | | | | | | | | | | | | |

*Source:* Reprinted with permission from the *Departmental Operating Manual,* Division of Continuing Studies, Columbus Campus, Indiana University-Purdue University at Indianapolis, ©1975.

The coordinator should pack all materials needed in addition to those described. Extra certificates and/or CEU records should be included for persons who register at the opening of the event or substitute for those previously registered. Supplies such as pencils, paper, Scotch tape, masking tape, marking pens, paper clips, and different colored papers should be included. A ballpoint pen is necessary for signing forms. All materials and supplies needed by the coordinator or secretary should be packed separately and marked "Materials for the Staff."

If audiovisual materials and equipment are to be taken by the staff, the equipment must be checked to be sure it is working properly, extra bulbs are included, and it is properly packed for safe transport. If a 16mm film is being used, an extra reel must be included.

Final preparations usually take place the day before the event. The coordinator and the secretary must schedule sufficient time and have space available to organize the materials and supplies.

## CONDUCTING THE EDUCATIONAL ACTIVITY

The day of the event, the coordinator and the secretary are responsible for being sure the room is set up properly, all equipment is in place and working, all materials are available, coffee is ready, and meals will be served as requested. Directions must be posted for the location of the activity. If a motel or hotel is being used, the room assignment should be posted on the activities board in the lobby. If a university or hospital is the site, room signs must be posted and persons at the information desk made aware of the location. Staff persons should wear nametags to help participants identify those in charge.

A registration table should be in an obvious location so each participant can obtain the materials and be checked in on the roster. The climate for the event is initiated with the first contact during registration. Participants should be made to feel comfortable, so the way they are greeted is important. The importance of the participant and the course or workshop are further emphasized when everything is well organized and registration moves smoothly. This assumes that all or the majority of the individuals have been handled through preregistration. If registration is to be handled at the event, additional staff persons must be available to assist with the process.

### The Introductory Phase

The coordinator is responsible for starting the session on time. As soon as the faculty person(s) arrive, the prepared materials should be reviewed, audiovisuals set up and tested, and the room arrangement checked.

The introductory phase of the session includes providing the participants with "housekeeping" information such as location of bathrooms, telephones, arrangements for meals, and so on. The objectives are stated along with a general overview of the schedule. Depending on the size of the group and the overall approach, the participants may be requested to introduce themselves and state their purpose in attending. This phase may be delayed, depending on whether a get-acquainted exercise and an objective-setting segment are included. The coordinator or a member of the planning committee may introduce the faculty.

During this introductory phase, the staff person or faculty establish the climate for the sessions. The structure of the event can determine its formality or informality. Participants need to know how questions and discussion will be handled, whether the instructor is to be interrupted at the time or whether all questions will be handled at one time later. The faculty should describe the content and methods to be used.

## How to Cope with Problems

Once the session has begun, the coordinator should be available to facilitate its smooth implementation and to handle any problems that may arise. There is always the potential for problems no matter how well the event has been planned. The bulb may go out in the audiovisual equipment, a participant or faculty member may become ill, or an emergency telephone call must be relayed to a participant or instructor.

More difficult problems may arise. What happens if at the last minute a faculty member cannot attend? It is important to have a backup plan or person. This is not as difficult to handle if several instructors are present. However, if one person is providing all or most of the instruction, this poses a major problem. If the department can afford to pay someone for preparation time and can locate an alternate who is willing to accept such a role, this will provide reasonable assurance that the event can be conducted as scheduled. If this is not possible, the only alternative is to cancel the session and/or reschedule at another time. If it is a series of classes or workshops to be conducted over a period of weeks, it may be easier to delay the start and extend the course an extra week or so. Another option is to cancel this session and increase the length of each other one if this is agreeable with the participants.

If several faculty members are being used, the coordinator is responsible for being sure they stay within their allotted time. If a speaker runs five to ten minutes past schedule, the coordinator should interrupt and indicate the time frame. This may be difficult, but it is essential for the event to achieve its stated objectives by ensuring that the other faculty members have time for their presentations. One way is to indicate that this speaker will be available during breaks or lunch if there are questions. Participants expect the sessions to be kept on schedule since they have allotted a certain amount of time to be present. If the schedule is not adhered to, many will leave at the time designated for the session to end. This creates frustration and dissatisfaction for participants, faculty, and the staff.

## After the Session

The coordinator should conclude the event by thanking faculty and participants, distributing certificates/CEU records, and collecting the completed evaluation/satisfaction index forms. This is a good time to make participants aware of future activities by having advance publicity available for distribution or announcement.

After the activity ends, the evaluations (satisfaction index) must be tabulated and summarized; thank-you letters sent to members of the planning committee and the faculty along with a copy of the evaluation summary; and a final check made to ensure that all forms for payment of faculty, rental(s), meals, and any other expenses have been processed. Reports of attendance are prepared and sent to the appropriate individual(s) or organizations and entered in the continuing education department record.

The last step is to be sure the permanent file for the event is complete and organized (Exhibit 8-8). The coordinator should complete an evaluation for future reference.

Beginning with the planning committee's identifying objectives, content, and potential resources for an educational activity on through its implementation, the staff coordinator devotes a great deal of time, skill, and energy to the project. To accomplish this, the coordinator must use good management skills, including organizing, planning, directing, and evaluating, and must be familiar with and follow all procedures established by the institution.

## Dealing with Cancellation

As noted, the implementation also should provide for actions in the event a workshop or class must be cancelled. Cancellation may occur as a result of (1) insufficient enrollment, (2) inability of the instructor(s) to keep their agreement to teach at the designated time, (3) weather conditions that make travel impossible for either the instructor(s) or participants.

The staff must decide whether to cancel if there is insufficient enrollment. In planning and budgeting for the event, the minimum number of registrations required to meet the budgeted costs is set. A registration deadline also

**Exhibit 8-8** Example of Checklist for Permanent File

PERMANENT FILE CHECKLIST FOR EDUCATIONAL OFFERING

I. Evaluation

   A. Summary of Participant Evaluation
   B. Instructor Evaluation Comments
   C. Staff Evaluation Comments

II. Facility

   A. Agreement/Reservation Form
   B. Copy of Payment Form
   C. Correspondence

III. Faculty

   A. Agreement for Teaching
   B. Vita
   C. Copy of Payroll Forms
   D. Correspondence

IV. Financial

   A. Budget/Cost Sheet
   B. Payment Form for:
      1. supplies
      2. books
      3. meals
      4. refreshments (coffee, doughnuts, soft drinks)
      5. other

V. Handout Materials/Forms

   A. Original Copy of Each Handout
   B. Forms Prepared for Offering:
      1. Computer Registration
      2. CEU Record
      3. Evaluation/Happiness Index
      4. Other (list)

VI. Offering Information

   A. Brochure
   B. Outline
   C. Schedule

VII. Participant Information

   A. Completed Registration Form
   B. Final Roster

VIII. Planning Committee

   A. List of Members
   B. Minutes
   C. Correspondence

*Source:* Reprinted with permission from the *Departmental Operating Manual,* Division of Continuing Studies, Columbus Campus, Indiana University-Purdue University at Indianapolis, ©1980.

is stated. In signing the teaching agreement, the instructor(s) are made aware of the minimum number required and the possibility of cancellation if this is not achieved. If the minimum number of registrations have not been received by the deadline, the coordinator decides to cancel the event after considering alternatives, including: (1) the number of registrations is so few that delaying a decision probably will not yield enough to conduct the course, (2) the number is so close to the minimum that delaying the decision for 24 to 48 hours may result in achieving the desired total, (3) the number is sufficient to cover all out-of-pocket or direct expenses but not any administrative costs, (4) the objectives and content are considered of such importance for those who have registered that the staff are willing to support the event out of funds from other activities.

Cancellation when the instructor reports an inability to keep the agreement depends largely on time. If time is available to locate another faculty member or if the defaulting instructor can provide a substitute, it may be possible to go ahead. If there is insufficient time for finding new instructors or the suggested substitutes are not acceptable, then the offering is cancelled and attempts are made to reschedule it at a later date with the same faculty. If rescheduling is possible, participants are notified and given the option of a refund if they are unable to attend at the new time.

Weather conditions present problems (particularly travel) for some areas of the country, especially in winter. If the continuing education program is located in a college or university, the department should be a part of the emergency closing procedures used for the other programs. The coordinator and secretary should have a list of instructors and their home telephone numbers in case they must be notified of cancellation because of weather. Similarly, a list of participants and their telephone numbers should be kept for courses being conducted over a number of weeks. If the weather is bad, the coordinator should make the decision to cancel as early as possible the morning of the event and, together with the secretary, notify all parties. The decision to reschedule is made later and participants notified, again with the option to attend at the new time or receive refunds.

In notifying the instructor(s) of a cancellation, the coordinator discusses the potential for rescheduling, if feasible. If the event is scheduled at an offsite location, the coordinator also notifies the facility. The secretary processes the cancellation notice to the appropriate persons or departments, including those responsible for facility scheduling if the event was to have been conducted in-house. Who in the departments should be notified is up to the particular organization but may include the director or dean of the department, the business office, the building and grounds department, and the bookstore. If meals were to have been provided, the appropriate person or department must be informed.

The secretary is responsible for processing refunds for all participants. Each organization should have a policy for this. The refunds should be made to the person if paid individually or to the organization if the payment was made by that entity.

---

## SUGGESTED READINGS

Clark, Carolyn Chambers. *The Nurse as Continuing Educator.* New York: Springer Publishing Co., 1979.

Davis, Larry, and McCallon, Earl. *Planning, Conducting and Evaluating Workshops.* Austin, Texas: Learning Concepts, 1974.

# Chapter 9

# Evaluation

Evaluation is an essential, and most often neglected, component of continuing education and staff development. Evaluation is essential to close the feedback loop—that is, to provide the department director with information necessary to improve the program. Indeed, evaluation can be viewed as essential if the program is to progress. Two aspects of evaluation with which the staff must be familiar are (1) evaluation of specific individual educational offerings and (2) evaluation of the total continuing education in nursing program.

The staff must be familiar with the terms used in evaluation, so it is appropriate to begin with a definition of evaluation as the means for determining the worth of an activity or program. Evaluation is an integral part of accountability, both to the agency that supports the program and to the participants who avail themselves of its services.

In the not too distant past, little or no attention was paid to evaluation in health care, including nursing. Changes in technology, politics, and economics placed responsibility on educational institutions to reexamine their role. At about the same time, there began a movement toward lifelong learning as the obsolescence of knowledge, especially in the health care professions, became more and more apparent. Groups such as legislators and funding agencies began asking for proof of the claims made by the programs as to what they would accomplish. Program directors coincidentally began to see the value of systematic evaluation.

Evaluation is used to demonstrate the worth of a program. It can describe a program's effectiveness and efficiency in meeting the needs it was designed to meet. Evaluation is used basically to find out if what is done is effective. The planning process begins with an assessment of the learner's needs to find out where to go; evaluation allows the staff to find out if the nurse got there.

Evaluation should be done consistently by the staff. Consistency here means that each course, class, or workshop will be evaluated at its completion, and the entire continuing education effort at least annually. The scope of the evaluation process should be determined on the basis of appropriateness for the program involved. Appropriateness can be assessed by determining the use to be made of the evaluative data; collection of extensive data is meaningless if they will not be used to improve the program. Evaluation is inappropriate if used only to fill file drawers with data. Appropriateness also is determined by the cost of the evaluation. If the department cannot afford to employ an external evaluator, then one should not be used.

## DATA COLLECTION TECHNIQUES

Techniques that the continuing education staff may find useful involve questionnaires, interviews, observation, tests and unobtrusive measures. Each of these techniques can be used singularly and in combination to provide the most effective means of evaluation. When used in combination, each technique will provide information that can be viewed in triangulation with any other data collected. Triangulation of data is the social science process of using multiple measures that overlap and don't have the same weaknesses.

The use of unobtrusive measures illustrates the technique of data triangulation. For example, in addition to testing knowledge obtained in a specific course, a continuing education staff member visits the library to determine how many of the references on the program bibliography were checked out by participants. This information then can be compared with test scores and perhaps even with observations of participants' performances at work. A description of each of the techniques and their application in continuing education and staff development will illustrate the methodology of evaluation.

### Questionnaires

A questionnaire is probably the most frequently used method of evaluation for an educational offering. Questionnaires generally are designed to assess the learner's happiness with the activity, asking questions such as "Did you like it?" or "Did you not like it?" This elicits feelings, perceptions, and subjective reactions to the course or workshop (Exhibit 9-1). While capable of obtaining useful information for program planners, these questionnaires are limited in the depth of information they provide, especially related to achievement of each course objective.

An expanded version can be designed to elicit the knowledge that the participants perceive they are acquiring in the course. One effective means is to list each of the behavioral objectives for the class, using a scale where 1 is low and 5 is high. The participants are asked to indicate the extent to

## Exhibit 9-1 Example of Evaluative Questionnaire

INDIANA STATEWIDE PLAN FOR CONTINUING EDUCATION IN NURSING

"EMERGENCY DEPARTMENT NURSING TODAY"

SATISFACTION QUESTIONNAIRE

PURPOSE:

To provide feedback from participants at specific intervals during the instruction period.

This questionnaire will be completed by participants at the end of each week of instruction. At the beginning of the second, third, fourth and fifth weeks of instruction opportunity will be provided for discussion of comments made and problems encountered in the application to the "back home" setting.

- Complete the following anonymously.

- Evaluate the first 5 days of the ER course: Sept. 28, Oct. 5, 12, 19, 26.

- Content in these sessions included:
      Expanded role of the nurse
      EMS Commission, structure
      Joint Commission & ANA Standard of Practice for ED's
      Physical Assessment
      Charting considerations
      History taking

- Specific comments are most helpful.

- Make comments about the Red Cross Course separately.

- Comments on shock will be made in subsequent questionnaire.

Circle the number representing your immediate impression about each statement. Use extreme numbers where your impression permits.

|  | Strongly Disagree | Disagree | Tend to Disagree | Tend to Agree | Agree | Strongly Agree |
|---|---|---|---|---|---|---|
| SECTION I |  |  |  |  |  |  |
| 1. The information presented was too elementary for me. | 1 | 2 | 3 | 4 | 5 | 6 |
| 2. Possible solutions to some of my problems were considered. | 1 | 2 | 3 | 4 | 5 | 6 |
| 3. We did not spend enough time relating theory to practice. | 1 | 2 | 3 | 4 | 5 | 6 |
| 4. The content presented was not applicable to my work. | 1 | 2 | 3 | 4 | 5 | 6 |
| 5. The purposes of the program were clear to me. | 1 | 2 | 3 | 4 | 5 | 6 |
| 6. I received few guidelines for future action. | 1 | 2 | 3 | 4 | 5 | 6 |

## Exhibit 9-1 continued

7. Programs such as this will con-
   tribute to changes in my practice.    1    2    3    4    5    6

8. The program objectives were <u>not</u>
   the objectives I expected.    1    2    3    4    5    6

9. The information presented was
   too advanced for me.    1    2    3    4    5    6

10. The material presented was
    valuable to me.    1    2    3    4    5    6

SECTION II

Be as specific as you can in responding to each statement.

1. Please list three specific things you plan to do as a result of your learning
   this week.

II. What specific things did you like <u>most</u> about this week of instruction?

III. What specific things did you like <u>least</u> about this week of instruction?

IV. Please make any other comments you care to.

*Source:* Reprinted by permission of Indiana Statewide Plan for Continuing Education in Nursing, Indianapolis, ©1976.

which they think they now can accomplish the behavior stated in each of the course objectives (Exhibit 9-2). A survey form using such a scale is easy to tabulate and interpret. Data collected in this fashion often are more useful than those that require extensive collation of essay-type comments. Summarization of these comments must be done cautiously so as not to lose their substance.

Other information that can be obtained through questionnaires that allows for evaluation of the content, process, and method of a workshop or course includes:

- to what extent the faculty or speakers were prepared and interesting

- to what extent the facilities were adequate

- to what extent there were opportunities for active participation by the nurses

- to what extent the organization of the course was consistent with its purpose

- how participants indicated they would use what they learned

- what the positive aspects of the activity were

- what the negative aspects were

- what improvements or modifications were suggested

- what suggestions were made for future workshops or courses

Elements related to any area of interest to the continuing education department can be included on a questionnaire. Problems arise, however, when questionnaires are too long and become unwieldy both for the participants and the person who must tabulate them. Evaluation questionnaires can be standardized for use in every educational activity, with an extra page added for the nurses to evaluate each specific class or course. Often specific questions such as "Was the faculty prepared and interesting?" will be answered also in the section "What did you like or dislike about the educational offering?"

## The Value of Experimentation

Experimenting with various evaluation questionnaires will permit the development of a form appropriate for specific program needs. At a minimum, evaluation questionnaires should ask for information related to what was learned, what will be done with what was learned, what could be improved, and what other events the nurses would like to attend or in what other subject areas they have educational needs. Repetitive questions or ones that do not

**Exhibit 9-2** Example of an Advanced Evaluative Questionnaire

INDIANA UNIVERSITY NORTHWEST CONTINUING NURSING EDUCATION PROGRAM

THE NURSES' ROLE IN PATIENT/FAMILY EDUCATION
May 16, 1980

HAPPINESS INDEX

1.  Please list your expectations for attending this workshop.

2.  Which of your expectations were met?

3.  In what ways did the workshop fail to satisfy your expectations?

4.  Please evaluate your personal degree of attainment of each workshop objective
    and check the appropriate boxes.

    Very Well                                                              Not
                                                                          at all

    a.  Identify the nurses' role in patient
        and family health education.
    b.  Compare the nursing process and the
        teaching-learning process.
    c.  Demonstrate selected teaching-learning
        theories for the adult patient in a
        role play situation.
    d.  Critique various teaching strategies used
        in patient education for appropriateness
        and effectiveness.

5.  I rate my degree of interest in this workshop as:

    HI                                        LO

6.  I rate the value received as:

    HI                                        LO

7.  The level of presentation was:

    _____Too theoretical--not enough "How to do it."
    _____Just the right blend of theory and practice.
    _____Too practical--not enough explanation of "why."

**Exhibit 9-2** continued

8. The method of presentation was:   (Check those that apply.)

_____Too much discussion, not enough lecture.
_____Too much lecture, not enough discussion.
_____Too much large group activity, not enough individual or small
       group activity.
_____Too much material covered.
_____Too little material covered.
_____About right.

9. My suggestions for modifying this workshop are:

10. My suggestions for other continuing nursing education courses are:

5/80MEM:mc

*Source:* Reprinted by permission of Continuing Nursing Education Program, Indiana University Northwest, Gary, Indiana, ©1980.

provide information that will be used should be avoided at all costs. Pilot testing of various types of evaluation questionnaires on the potential audience can provide information that may lead to revisions or modification and thus ultimately to a more effective form without sacrificing useful data. Analyzing a proposed evaluation form with a panel of experts in continuing education can yield useful suggestions for revisions or modifications.

### Improving Acceptance of the Form

Participants may be reluctant to complete evaluation forms at the conclusion of a course. Many times they are eager to leave for home. If the course runs over the time allotted, time for the evaluation is minimized. Various methods can help ensure a good completion rate. One way is to tell the nurses at the beginning of the event, when reviewing the agenda for the day, that evaluation time has been set aside so they can share their reactions with the program developers. The need for each nurse to complete the form must be stressed, and what will be done with the information they provide must be explained. They often indicate that they feel the evaluations don't make any difference; knowing that evaluation is viewed as an essential component of the course can dispel this notion. If attendance certificates are awarded, the participants can be handed their certificates in "exchange" for the completed evaluation forms. Similarly, evaluations can be "exchanged" for continuing education unit (CEU) records (assuming that CEU will be awarded upon completion of the course).

In a staff development department of an institution where most of the course participants are employees of the institution, evaluation forms can be tabulated and a summary posted on the bulletin board. If the nurses' evaluations indicated that changes are needed in the course, the program planner can note on the summary what will be changed. This proves to the nurses beyond a doubt that the evaluation information they provided is indeed used.

This example is limited to instances where most of the participants are from one health care institution. When many come from other institutions, the cost of mailing evaluation summaries to each participant may be prohibitive, but efforts can be made to let them know how the information they provided was used.

One effective method is to include comments from previous evaluations in publicity for a course when it is repeated. Such promotional material often is sent to past participants, who may recognize a comment they made; this can reinforce what was said about the use made of the evaluations. Participants in repeat sessions can be told at the outset what changes have been made as a result of previous evaluations. Such techniques encourage word-of-mouth dissemination of exactly the information the planners want spread around—that is, that evaluation is important to them and, by implication, should be important to the participants.

There are techniques to ensure that nurses complete the evaluation form. Standardized forms may become boring to repeat students. Unless printing is a problem, in that vast quantities of evaluation forms must be printed for use over a long period, varying the color and size of the paper can help. Using 5″ × 8″ index cards instead of 8½″ × 11″ paper can add variety. If the educational offering is composed of a number of course sessions rather than a one-day format, an index card can be used for each class and the overall evaluation can be a composite of these individual evaluations. Since only evaluation summaries need be filed, the originals can be discarded when the summary is completed.

Evaluation questionnaires always should be completed anonymously, even though this can pose problems if follow-ups are desired. (Techniques for handling this are discussed later in this chapter.)

## Interviews

Interviewing is a useful means of obtaining evaluative information. Interviews are costlier and more time consuming than questionnaires. They can provide information of more value than that obtained by questionnaires, depending on the degree to which the planners can define exactly what they want to know and what the possible range of answers might be. Questionnaires do not allow for formulation of follow-up queries nor for clarification of answers. Interview responses can be triangulated with information obtained from questionnaires. Triangulation of data might well be an essential component of a decision to change a course or workshop, to verify that the new steps are appropriate, or when the participant-evaluators deem modifications necessary but the planner is uncertain what specific ones would improve the offering.

To obtain the most useful information, the interviewer probably will find a standardized list of questions most helpful. A standardized interview is one in which precisely the same information is collected from a number of respondents. This information can be compared more easily than that from a nonstandardized interview. Variations in answers thus are due to differences in respondents rather than in the questions.

A scheduled interview should be used, with the questions and the order in which they are to be asked specified in advance.

## Observation

Observation is a useful method of evaluation both in the learning setting and the work environment. If learning skills form a component of the course, a skills checklist (Exhibit 9-3) is valuable for recording observations. This form then can be completed at the work station to determine the extent that the classroom learning was transferred to the job. Observation requires skills beyond merely glancing around. The observer needs to be told specifically what is to be scrutinized. Observation guides can be developed so that individuals other than the staff can collect data. Triangulation of data from interviews can be compared with information obtained from observation if, for instance, a participant in a skills workshop is asked about what was learned and how it can be applied. The skills checklist could confirm or contradict what was said in the interview.

## Tests

If tests are to be effective as a means of evaluation, they must be reliable and valid. (Those elements are discussed in detail in the section of this chapter on analysis of evaluative data.)

Tests should be constructed after the course objectives have been specified. The individual constructing the test selects questions compatible with the anticipated results of the classes. The questions can be those where the correct answer is either recognized or constructed. Recognition items are simpler to design and can be scored more easily and more objectively than those in which the learner must construct the response. In the latter, the test designer must provide precisely specified criteria by which the responses will be rated.

Tests should be constructed so they are easy to administer. Directions must be clear and simple, so that time is not spent in explanations, and they must be reasonable in length. A pretest or posttest should take no longer than half an hour, and a final examination not more than one hour.

If appropriately constructed, tests can ascertain level of cognition, not just a replay of facts. Pretests and posttests can be used to determine the extent to which the participants learned what they were supposed to learn.

Written tests constitute a good way of measuring learning when used in a pretest and posttest format, but unfortunately, may not be readily acceptable to most adults. Many adults have experienced "test anxiety" that can have an adverse effect even in a relatively nonthreatening environment such as a continuing education course. This anxiety can be reduced by resorting to tests only when other methods of evaluation are not feasible or telling participants that the scores will not be used to determine whether they pass, but to help them decide better what they need to learn.

Allowing the students to take the test anonymously can reduce anxiety but this may not provide information needed by the faculty or staff. Learners can be asked to record their pretest and posttest scores on their evaluation forms. The evaluations also are anonymous, but mean scores can be calculated from

**Exhibit 9-3 Example of an Educational Skills Checklist**

EMERGENCY DEPARTMENT NURSING TODAY

CHECKLIST OF SKILLS

NAME _____

| Skills | Observe | Simulation | Performance | Comments |
|---|---|---|---|---|
| II. Assessment | | | | |
| 1. Physical exam | | | | |
|   a. observation | | | | |
|   b. palpation | | | | |
|   c. percussion | | | | |
|   d. auscultation | | | | |
| 2. Elicit history | | | | |
|   a. interviewing skills | | | | |
|   b. accident/sudden illness | | | | |
|   c. health history | | | | |
|   d. family exam | | | | |
| 3. Record exam | | | | |
| 4. Record history | | | | |
| I. Technique | | | | |
| 1. Immobilize extremity | | | | |
| 2. Moving patients | | | | |
| 3. Aseptic technique | | | | |
| 4. Obtain cultures | | | | |
| 5. Suture removal | | | | |

MODULE I

MODULE II

**Exhibit 9-3 continued**

EMERGENCY DEPARTMENT NURSING TODAY

CHECKLIST OF SKILLS

Page Two

| Skills | Observe | Simulation | Performance | Comments |
|---|---|---|---|---|
| **MODULE II (CONT'D)** | | | | |
| 6. Sterile technique | | | | |
| 7. Veno puncture | | | | |
| 8. Insertion of indwelling I.V. | | | | |
| 9. Arterial puncture | | | | |
| 10. Male catheters | | | | |
| 11. Record skills | | | | |
| I. Respiratory | | | | |
| 1. Assess the respiratory status | | | | |
| 2. Suction | | | | |
| a. oral | | | | |
| b. nasal | | | | |
| c. tracheostomy | | | | |
| d. endotracheal | | | | |
| 3. Mouth-to mouth | | | | |
| 4. Manual resuscitation | | | | |
| 5. Using respirators | | | | |
| 6. Assist tracheostomy | | | | |
| 7. Intubation | | | | |
| a. assist | | | | |
| **MODULE III** | | | | |

EMERGENCY DEPARTMENT NURSING TODAY

CHECKLIST OF SKILLS

Page Three

| Skills | Observe | Simulation | Performance | Comments |
|---|---|---|---|---|
| b. perform | | | | |
| 8. Administer oxygen/humidity | | | | |
| 9. Record respiratory status | | | | |
| II. Cardiovascular | | | | |
| 1. Interpret EKG-evaluate EKG rhythm strip | | | | |
| 2. Assess cardiovascular status | | | | |
| 3. Cardiac instrumentation | | | | |
| a. EKG's/hookup & monitor | | | | |
| b. defibrillation | | | | |
| c. cardiac pacing | | | | |
| 4. Cardiopulmonary resuscitation | | | | |
| 5. Record cardiovascular status | | | | |
| III. Shock | | | | |
| 1. Initiate, maintain IV | | | | |
| 2. Regulate Fluids | | | | |
| 3. Electrolytes and medication | | | | |
| 4. Open airway-circulation | | | | |
| 5. Regulate body temperature | | | | |
| 6. Psychosocial support | | | | |

MODULE III (CONT'D)

*Source:* Reprinted by permission of Indiana Statewide Plan for Continuing Education in Nursing, Indianapolis, ©1976.

the two sets of numbers. Changing the name from pretest or posttest to self-assessment can help to reduce anxiety.

Various other techniques can be used to test learning. Films can be run without the accompanying sound to test observation. Students can be asked to identify what they saw in the film and what they would do about what they saw. The film could be run at the beginning of the course and again at the end so that the differences in observation or actions could be compared to determine whether learning took place.

Acquisition of skills is easier to test using a performance checklist similar to that described in the previous section on observation. This checklist can be used for pretests and posttests. Participants can be asked how many of the skills they are able to perform at the beginning and end of the course, and the number compared, with an actual demonstration to verify that they can do what they say they can.

Simulation games are useful not only as a teaching strategy but also as an evaluative means. A simulation game can be designed with two alternate forms—a pretest and a posttest—and the results compared.

Case studies or vignettes can be used to describe situations to which the learner must respond in some specified manner. Similar case studies can be presented at the beginning and end of a course and the results compared in pretests and posttests.

## Unobtrusive Measures

Unobtrusive measures generally are used to supplement other forms of evaluation. Triangulation of information from unobtrusive measures with data from other forms of evaluation is particularly valuable. Unobtrusive measures, as described by Webb, refer to measures that do not require the cooperation of a respondent and that do not themselves contaminate the response, such as physical evidence, archives, and observations.[1] Reviews of charting or inspections of nursing audits are unobtrusive measures, as are wear on textbook pages, use of references, and scratch pad consumption. Taken alone, these may not be significant but in combination with data from other evaluative methods may be of considerable use.

### NEGATIVE FEEDBACK

The evaluation process always provides some negative feedback for the program planner. Unless the planner is prepared for this, the results can be devastating for one who has expended much time and effort to produce the perfect educational offering, only to find that some persons didn't like it. In reviewing evaluations, the continuing education staff must exercise judgment about what to do with negative feedback, based on the fact that some people always will be dissatisfied, and some things can't be changed. Negative comments may be related to the physical setting for the course. That environment should be as conducive to learning as possible, but occasionally there will be heating or ventilation problems that cannot be cured. Participants' negative comments about these factors should merely be accepted. If the environment can be changed, then it should be; if not, it merely should be accepted as one of the factors about which nothing can be done. The staff must exercise judgment as to whether the negative comments are unwarranted. If comments involve a situation beyond the control of the planners but permeate the participants' evaluations, there may be a need to take action beyond merely accepting or ignoring the remarks. For example, if a class is held in a facility that does not serve meals or coffee, so that participants must go outside for them, the staff may want to summarize the evaluations, add an explanation about that situation, and mail these materials to all the participants. While this can be costly, such a good-will effort may induce the nurses to return for future courses. The explanation should state what will be done in the future, such as catering coffee breaks and meals.

Comments on changes in the workshop or course should be viewed on the basis of what realistically can be done. Once all possible changes are made, the activity can be repeated, and the evaluations compared to see if moves made a difference.

## FOLLOW-UP EVALUATION

Follow-up evaluation can be used to determine how well the nurses could use what they learned. Unfortunately, because something was learned cognitively that does not mean it will be applied on the job. Participants' perceptions of their ability to implement what they learned may not be accurate.

The follow-up evaluation can be a questionnaire that asks the nurse to describe what was learned in class and what was applied on the job. The questionnaire should be constructed according to the methods described earlier in this chapter.

Interviews can be used for follow-up evaluation. They should follow the guidelines for the interview method of data collection discussed earlier. They can be conducted in person or by telephone with a random sample of the participants. Cost and time considerations may make this less desirable than other methods.

Nursing audits are effective as follow-up evaluations that also can indicate additional educational needs. If nursing audits were used to determine the need for a specific course, then a review after a specific time since the class ended is the evaluative method of choice.

## Difficulties

There are two major difficulties associated with follow-up evaluation: (1) anonymity and (2) low return rate.

Evaluations should always be completed anonymously. If, however, participants are asked to indicate what they will do with what they learned, with a follow-up in six months to determine if they actually did so, then that part of the evaluation cannot be anonymous or follow-up would be impossible. The questions that will be used in the follow-up evaluation should be listed on a separate sheet of paper. This paper also asks for the respondent's name and address. The respondent is then identified only on the follow-up portion of the evaluation. The remainder of the evaluative questions are answered anonymously. Separating out the follow-up question will make the participants aware that such an evaluation will take place.

As for the notoriously small return of completed evaluation forms, this rate generally can be improved somewhat by the inclusion of a stamped, self-addressed envelope with the follow-up questionnaire, but this is not guaranteed to produce a dramatic improvement. Mail or telephone reminders may prod those who failed to return their forms. Coding the questionnaires in some manner may help the evaluator identify those who did not return them. There is·the chance that the respondent will discern that the questionnaire is coded, so that may reduce the return rate. If there is to be follow-up of nonreturned forms, the respondents should be informed. If follow-up is not possible because of cost or other factors, informing respondents may encourage some to return forms they might not have otherwise.

Keeping follow-up questionnaires simple will enhance the return rate. For example, the form can be constructed to consist of only four questions: (1) These are the three things you said you would do as a result of the educational activity you attended (identify it). To what extent were you able to do what you said you would do? (2) What were the factors that helped you do what you said you would? (3) What were the factors that hindered you from doing this? (4) How could the activity have helped you better?

Follow-up evaluation may not serve its intended purpose; in that case, it's better not to attempt it just because it "should be done."

## USE OF EVALUATIONS

Evaluation data, in addition to pointing out needed changes in the course, can indicate future educational requirements and thus facilitate planning. Evaluations should be shared with the course planners, the faculty, and the participants to the extent that this is feasible. Evaluation data are useful in the compilation of reports. Accreditation or approval of individual activities and the total continuing education program may require that specific use be made of evaluative methods and data (Chapter 10).

Recordkeeping space may not permit retaining all of the nurses' evaluations; once these are summarized, the originals can be destroyed and only the summary maintained on file. If comments on the forms are summarized, several of the original responses can be kept with the summary to indicate the accuracy with which the remarks were recapitulated.

## PROGRAM EVALUATION

Another major component of the continuing education staff's responsibility is program evaluation. At least annually, the program's worth to the institution and to the audience it serves should be evaluated. The data gathering techniques used in program evaluation are those described earlier in this chapter: questionnaires, interviews, observation, tests, and unobtrusive measures. Program evaluation methods vary from the simple to the complex. Perhaps the simplest is for a group of individuals to review the stated objectives and determine the extent to which they have been reached in the past year. This is referred to as discrepancy evaluation because it reveals the differences between program plans and actual achievements.

For example, the group responsible for evaluating a hospital staff development department could consist of persons in the department, the director of nursing, supervisory personnel, and staff nurses. This group would meet and review the evidence of results provided by the department director. An objective such as "To teach all hospital personnel the technique of cardiopulmonary resuscitation (CPR)" could be measured easily by reviewing CPR course attendance statistics in comparison with personnel department statistics on the number of hospital employees.

Given an internal committee of evaluators, it is best because of vested interest for the continuing education representative to serve as the facilitator of the evaluative process rather than as a member of the committee. As a facilitator, this individual would provide information to the committee and remain available to respond to questions and obtain additional data as required. The committee's report then becomes the evaluation of the department.

The department director may want to employ someone to assist with the evaluation. An external evaluator has the advantage of being able to see something in the situation from an objective viewpoint that an internal person may not discern because of close involvement in the program. Because of the staff person's familiarity with the program being evaluated, the insider is aware of subtleties that the external evaluator may overlook. Thus, working together, the two provide an effective combination of viewpoints. They share responsibility for the evaluation and together they select the method to be used.

## Evaluation Models

Evaluation models generally fall into four types, based on the kinds of decisions to be made:

1. *Context* evaluation helps in making planning decisions for a continuing program. Decisions have to be made in the context of the organizational structure and the goals and objectives of the program. Discrepancy evaluation is in the category of context evaluation. After the evaluation is completed, decisions can be made that will reduce discrepancies between what is planned and what actually occurs.
2. *Input* evaluation aids in decision making that results in the putting-into-action of the goals of the program. It provides information about what means and resources are necessary to meet the ends (goals) of the program. Such an evaluation may result in the conclusion that the goals are unrealistic or unattainable.
3. *Process* evaluation assists in the everyday decision making of program directors, involving such factors as interpersonal relationships, performance of staff, and facilities. Process evaluation also records events through regular data collection to document occurrences throughout the life of a program.
4. *Product* evaluation measures and interprets program achievements— whether the objectives have been attained. This method generally is reserved for evaluation at the end of a program but can be used during the course of an activity to provide quality control. Product evaluation can be used in decision making as to whether to terminate a program, continue funding, or make modifications.

An evaluation method that encompasses all four types is Stufflebeam's Content, Input, Process, Product (CIPP) model.[2] A goal-free evaluation is designed by Scriven.[3] This model has as a focus the actual, not the intended, effects of a program; these may differ considerably. The emphasis on goals, according to Scriven, is appropriate in the evaluation of a proposal for a program but not of the process or the end product. In this model, data are collected without knowledge or reference to the program goals. The goals can be inferred from the actual effects of the program, but this is not a necessary step with this model. The result of the use of goal-free evaluation is a direct assessment of a program's worth.

Any one of several other models such as those described by Worthen and Sanders[4] can be selected to evaluate a particular continuing education program.

## Use of a Consultant

The program director may wish to employ a consultant to conduct the evaluation. In that case, the consultant decides which model and data gathering techniques are to be used and communicates this to the program director.

The director then serves only to provide the information necessary to conduct the process but does not participate as an internal evaluator. This method probably is the most objective but can cause misinterpretation of data by the evaluator, who may not be intimately familiar with the program. This method frees the director from a substantial amount of work, however, and may be more feasible in certain situations.

The consultant should be selected on the basis of expertise in program evaluation. As an external appraiser, the consultant needs primarily to be familiar with the evaluation process rather than with the content of the specific program under study. That is, the evaluator does not need to be knowledgeable about the health care professions in order to analyze the effectiveness of a continuing education program in nursing. An evaluator with a peripheral familiarity of the subject, of course, may be more comfortable in the job, and the department director may select the individual with this in mind.

If a consultant is being hired, the terms of the evaluation should be negotiated before an agreement is signed to avoid later misunderstandings. These terms should include the evaluator's fee and method of payment—for example, at the end of the evaluation, or in partial payments such as one-third at the start, one-third on submission of a rough draft report, and one-third at the end of the process. Details such as what data are to be gathered, and how, can be negotiated on a verbal basis and do not necessarily need to be part of the written agreement.

The department director may choose to evaluate the program. This approach is the most subjective, of course, but the results can be presented in light of that factor and readers forewarned to interpret the outcome accordingly. If the director decides to go it alone, any appropriate evaluation model can be selected. If possible, the director should seek help from an individual with some expertise in evaluation in order to best implement the selected model. If this is not possible, a group of individuals involved in the program being evaluated most likely can be of assistance and also aid in ameliorating the attendant subjectivity. If an advisory committee has been established for the continuing education program, this may be the appropriate group to assist with the evaluation.

Many decisions about evaluation depend upon the use to be made of the results. If the evaluation is being done primarily to justify continuing (or increased) funding, subjectivity had better be minimized. On the other hand, if it is primarily for an accrediting or approval body, a costly, sophisticated evaluation probably is not necessary or even desirable. Evaluation should be useful in determining future directions for the program; an evaluation that does not supply some useful guidelines for the future is not worth the time and effort. Many evaluations that slumber on dusty shelves are a result of an overly ambitious design where a plethora of new data were gathered, analyzed, and described for the wrong reasons, which led to less than useful results.

## Discomfort and Anxiety

Finally, a word about the discomfort that may be felt by continuing education staff members as they participate in the evaluation of their program. This discomfort is hardly avoidable since it is their program that is under scrutiny and might be found seriously lacking in some essential area. Some of this anxiety may be a result of lack of knowledge about the evaluative process. This anxiety can be ameliorated by a review of the many materials readily available to acquaint novices with educational evaluation.

The anxiety over being held accountable for the worth of the program is more difficult to cope with. No evaluation, if done properly, will reveal perfection, with no improvement or change necessary. That is an unrealistic expectation. Although staff members may feel perfectly comfortable with the results of the evaluation, they may not be as comfortable sharing them with others, particularly when the deficiencies identified seem glaring.

One technique for minimizing the effects of others' criticisms is to append to the report the department director's acceptance of the recommendations for improvement and some indication of how this executive plans to implement them. This is done best in a nondefensive manner without a lot of justification as to why things are as they are. It may be well to write a draft of this appendix and ask several colleagues to review and comment on it and, more importantly, on the tone of the writing. Everyone is defensive when what they are involved in is attacked, but in this instance a defensive posture will not accomplish anything.

## ANALYSIS OF EVALUATIVE DATA

Instruments used for evaluation must have two characteristics: reliability and validity. All of the instruments used, whether questionnaires or tests, must be both reliable and valid.

## Reliability

Reliability refers to the consistency with which the instrument will measure a subject; that is, the extent to which the evaluation tool will consistently measure the same characteristic over time. This is compounded in difficulty by the fact that what is being evaluated may itself be an unstable characteristic and not be capable of being measured over time. For purposes of this discussion, however, the characteristics being measured are considered to be stable. A reliable instrument, then, is one that provides a stable, consistent measurement time after time, over an extended period.

Reliability is expressed in statistical terms as a coefficient of correlation—that is, the relationship of two sets of scores or measures.

Coefficients of correlation range from $+1.00$ through $0.0$ to $-1.00$. If the coefficient is $+1.00$, there is a perfect positive relationship, so that as one score increases, the other will rise correspondingly. A coefficient of $-1.00$ also is a perfect correlation, but a negative one, so that as one score increases, the other will decrease. A coefficient of $0.0$ indicates that there is no relationship present between the two variables, other than what might exist by chance. The closer the coefficient is to either $+1.00$ or to $-1.00$, the stronger the relationship is between the two sets of scores.

The strength of the relationship is expressed numerically; that is, coefficients of correlation of $+.85$ and $-.85$ are equally strong, only with different directions—one positive and one negative. If the relationship is strong, the correlation will be close to either $+1.00$ or $-1.00$, which indicates that the instrument used in the measurement is reliable. The assumption is that the instrument was stable over time, no matter how many times it was applied. The acceptability of the finding of evaluative procedures often is based on the extent to which the instruments or procedures used were reliable. Therefore, the continuing education director would do well to understand and be able to use statistical methods in order to demonstrate the reliability of the evaluation instruments and procedures.

There are several ways to obtain coefficients of correlation to demonstrate reliability. Many can be obtained without involvement of a statistician or computer analysis. However, a computer does simplify data analysis. When collected data are to be analyzed by computer, they should be put onto computer cards directly whenever possible. If that is not possible, they can be transferred to computer cards by keypunch operators.

Reliability can be measured by the *test-retest* method: the same instrument, such as a test or questionnaire, is given to a group of individuals on two different occasions, usually about a week apart. The correlation between their scores on the first and second occasions is computed. The computation can take the form of a coefficient of correlation or a percentage of agreement.

Some items on the instrument may not be appropriate for calculating a coefficient of correlation. In that case, a percentage of agreement can be computed. This is a simpler method than a correlation coefficient and is done easily with a hand calculator.

The test-retest method is useful when attempting to determine the reliability of instruments that measure skill, such as a clinical performance checklist, but is less effective for those that attempt to measure knowledge, such as with multiple choice or true-false tests, because the participants may remember what they marked on the first occasion and respond the same way on the second. The reliability of the instrument then may appear better than it actually is. Attitudes and opinions may change over time, even over one week, so that the test-retest method is not appropriate for determining the reliability of instruments that measure attitudes or opinions, either.

Another way to measure reliability is to use *alternate* or *parallel* forms of the same test. The same group of individuals completes both forms of the test and the scores are correlated to determine reliability. The same material is covered in each of the alternate forms but the questions are different on each. This method overcomes the problem of the individual's ability to remember an answer from one testing occasion to another, as can occur with the test-retest technique.

A method similar to the alternate forms is the *split-half* method, in which one test is divided into halves that are equal in number of questions, difficulty, and so on. The tests can be divided by assigning odd-numbered questions to one half and even-numbered questions to the other. Individuals may complete either or both halves. The coefficient of correlation is calculated on the basis of the scores on the two halves.

Reliability is a concept that has been explored especially in relation to tests, but instruments that are used to rate or observe also can be tested for their reliability, generally using the percentage of agreement method. Correlations of sets of observation or rating forms can be calculated to determine reliability. More sophisticated methods of determining reliability can be attempted with assistance from a statistician or someone knowledgeable about computers and data analysis.

## Validity

Validity is the other characteristic that evaluative instruments or procedures must possess. It is defined as the extent to which an instrument measures what it is intended to measure. Validity is applicable to the tests, questionnaires, survey forms, observations, and ratings used in evaluation of continuing education. It also is a component of the design chosen by the program director for evaluating projects. In that instance, validity refers primarily to how well the evaluation's conclusions can be interpreted and generalized (generalization is important so evaluative conclusions are not situation specific but can be applied to different settings in different subjects or both). These two aspects of validity are interrelated, for useful conclusions about the effectiveness of a program cannot be drawn from evaluation designs that involve poor instruments, nor can the best of measures salvage a poor design.

Although most definitions of the concept concern the validity of the instrument itself, the one most useful to the program director is that which describes the validity of the inferences drawn from the results of the test, questionnaire, rating, or observation. The most critical inferences drawn from evaluative data by the program director or others involve whether a desired outcome was attained, such as whether the nurses achieved the objectives of a course or whether the program accomplished its goals to the extent it forecast. Three conceptions of validity have the most use to program directors:

1. *Construct* validity refers to the extent to which scores on a measure will allow inferences to be drawn about underlying traits. Construct validity usually is estimated from correlations of the measure with others. Scores on the instrument should show a significant relationship to those on others that measure the same trait and should show no significant relationship to results on unrelated measures. Another method would be to use a group of independent raters to measure the behavior in situations in which the trait is in operation.

2. *Content* validity refers to the degree to which the instrument measures what is being studied. The content of the instrument must be identical to what is being measured. A questionnaire about continuing education participation must not measure attitudes toward continuing education instead. The determination about content validity may be made by a single individual—usually the person who designed the instrument. A method that will ensure a greater degree of validity is to have the instrument reviewed by a panel of experts who will make the determination about its content. The experts should be individuals who are involved in the field under study. In the case of the questionnaire about participation in continuing education, others in the field could be used as members of the panel of experts. In instruments being prepared to test knowledge of certain subjects, nurses and others involved in that area could be members of the panel. Items in the draft questionnaire or test being reviewed that do not relate to what is being studied, measured, or tested should be eliminated from the final product.

3. *Face* validity refers to the degree to which the investigator or others determine that an instrument is valid on its face. There is a high degree of subjectivity related to the assessment of validity using this method

so that, again, the use of a group rather than an individual is preferable. This is not a method that requires much expertise or time but probably is the least preferable way to determine validity.

There are many other descriptions of assessment of the validity of a measure. Several of the more common types are *concurrent, predictive, criterion-related,* and *convergent* validity. The usual indicators of validity are coefficients of correlation so that a continuing education program director who is familiar and comfortable with calculating these will have little difficulty in assessing the instruments being evaluated. Other methods of determining validity can be explored if the program director is interested. There are many textbooks in statistics or evaluation and research methodology that can be of use to the director who wishes to go beyond the basic methods described here. (See Suggested Readings at the end of this chapter.)

## Validity in Program Evaluation

In using the concept of validity related to the design for program evaluation, the director is concerned primarily with the aspects being interpreted and generalized. The evaluative process of a continuing education program requires some kind of measurement or collection of data. The conditions under which that measurement is made or those data are collected constitute the design of the evaluation. Any evaluation design is adequate if the results can be interpreted and if the conclusions can be generalized. The question to be asked is whether the findings could be attributed to factors other than the program being evaluated. For example, the outcome of an evaluation of a program might be the result of:

1. local events (an upsurge of feminism causes nurses to become more assertive, rather than increased assertiveness being the result of their attending a continuing education workshop on assertiveness);
2. instability of the measurement instruments;
3. variations in the data collection (different people collecting data differently); or
4. the effects of initial measures on later ones (as in pretests and posttests).

If the findings of an appraisal can be attributed to causes other than the program itself, the evaluation design is not a valid one—the design is analyzing factors other than those it should be measuring.

The evaluator of a continuing education program also is interested in how well the conclusions can be generalized. The key question here is whether there is anything about the chosen design that would make it inappropriate to assume that similar effects might be found if it were applied to evaluate a similar program. For example, if the design is being applied to a continuing education program in a college or university, are the results likely to be found in the next town or state in which the same evaluation might be used in a campus nursing program? If the participants studied are not similar to the population of those in the parallel continuing education program, the conclusions drawn about those in the first group cannot be generalized. As an example, if the evaluation encompasses multiple aspects of the program, then the conclusions may not be relevant to a situation where only some of those factors exist.

## STATISTICAL TECHNIQUES

In any evaluation effort, there will be data collected that need to be analyzed. One method of data analysis that can be understood by anyone looking at the results is to use some basic statistical analysis. Data analyzed statistically have the same meaning to everyone who tries to interpret that information; that is, the results are consistently consistent. Statistics are a way of organizing and describing data so that they can be understood by everyone. Several statistical techniques should be included in every continuing education program director's repertoire: calculation of a frequency count, mean, median, and correlation of coefficient.

### Frequency Count

A frequency count is a tabulation of the number of times a certain score or other index occurs. For example, *10* students received a passing score on the pretest, or *43* nurses indicated they participated in one or more continuing education courses last year.

## Mean

A mean is an average of all the scores (the total of all the scores divided by the number of tests). For example, the scores for a pretest and posttest in a continuing education course on emergency lifesaving techniques were:

**MEAN**

| Participant | Pretest Scores | Posttest Scores |
|:-----------:|:--------------:|:---------------:|
| 1 | 14 | 17 |
| 2 | 24 | 22 |
| 3 | 20 | 21 |
| 4 | 18 | 16 |
| 5 | 11 | 10 |

**MEAN** continued

| Participant | Pretest Scores | Posttest Scores |
|:-----------:|:--------------:|:---------------:|
| 6 | 12 | 11 |
| 7 | 23 | 15 |
| 8 | 15 | 18 |
| 9 | 8 | 9 |
| 10 | 10 | 10 |
| | 155 | 149 |

mean: 155 ÷ 10 = 15.5                    mean: 149 ÷ 10 = 14.9

## Median

The median is the number above which half of all the cases in a sample fall and below which half of the cases fall. For example, in the previous illustration of pretests and posttests, the scores are arranged in order from highest to lowest and the middle number then is found.

**MEDIAN**

| Pretest | Posttest |
|:-------:|:--------:|
| 24 | 22 |
| 23 | 21 |
| 20 | 18 |
| 18 | 17 |
| 15 | 16 |
| 14 | 15 |
| 12 | 11 |
| 11 | 10 |
| 10 | 10 |
| 8 | 9 |

When there is an even number of cases, such as with this example of 10 pretest and posttest scores, the middle number or median is between two scores. The usual procedure is to call the halfway point the median; for example, the median for the pretest is 14.5 and for the posttest is 15.5.

## Coefficient of Correlation

The purpose of a coefficient of correlation is to express the strength or intensity of the relationship between two measures. One fairly simple way of calculating this without benefit of a computer is a Spearman rank correlation, which expresses in statistical terms the strength of a relationship between two measures. This method is applicable particularly when calculating data from 30 or fewer cases, otherwise it becomes too cumbersome.

In an example where there are alternate forms of a test (form A and form B) and both were given to each of ten participants in a continuing education class, five participants took the form A test followed by form B, and five in reverse order. The participants were assigned randomly to each of the two ways of taking the test (Exhibit 9-4).

The formula for calculating a Spearman rank order correlation is as follows:

$$\text{rho} = 1 - \frac{6 \, \Sigma \, D^2}{N \, (N^2 - 1)}$$

In this formula, rho is the coefficient of correlation, D is the difference in rank for each person, and N is the number of participants.

The steps to be followed in calculating the coefficient of correlation are:

1. Assign a rank (in this instance 1 through 10) to the scores on test A, giving the highest rank (1) to the highest score.
2. Assign a rank from 1 through 10 to the scores on test B, giving the highest rank (1) to the highest score.
3. Determine the difference in the participant's rank on test A and on test B; that figure is D.
4. Square D and enter the result in the column headed $D^2$.
5. Enter the appropriate numbers into the formula and solve the problem.

## SUMMARY

The continuing education program director must have a basic level of familiarity with statistical analysis. More important is the ability to interpret statistical data. There are a variety of resources available for increased learning of which the program director should take advantage.

The director also should be aware of the resources available to help identify appropriate statistical methods and data analysis. Local colleges and universities with computer centers offer assistance in instrument design and in data collection, analysis, and interpretation. Many large hospitals have departments devoted solely to research in which there are individuals who can help in evaluation design and in analysis of evaluative data.

**Exhibit 9-4** Sample Coefficient of Correlation

### SPEARMAN RANK DIFFERENCE METHOD

| Partic-ipant | Test Form A | Test Form B | Rank Form A $R_A$ | Rank Form B $R_B$ | Differ-ence D | Square of the Difference $D^2$ |
|---|---|---|---|---|---|---|
| 1 | 14 | 17 | 6 | 4 | 2 | 4 |
| 2 | 24 | 22 | 1 | 1 | 0 | 0 |
| 3 | 20 | 21 | 3 | 2 | 1 | 1 |
| 4 | 18 | 16 | 4 | 5 | 1 | 1 |
| 5 | 11 | 10 | 8 | 8.5 | .5 | .25 |
| 6 | 12 | 11 | 7 | 7 | 0 | 0 |
| 7 | 23 | 15 | 2 | 6 | 4 | 16 |
| 8 | 15 | 18 | 5 | 3 | 2 | 4 |
| 9 | 8 | 9 | 10 | 10 | 0 | 0 |
| 10 | 10 | 10 | 9 | 8.5 | .5 | .25 |
| | | | | | | 26.5 |

$$rho = 1 \frac{- 6 \times 26.5}{10 (10^2 - 1)}$$

$$rho = 1 \frac{- 159}{999}$$

$$rho = 1 - .159$$

$$rho = +.84$$

## NOTES

1. E. Webb, Donald Campbell, Richard Schwartz, Lee Schmidt, *Unobtrusive Measures: Non-reactive Research in the Social Sciences* (Chicago: Rand McNally, 1966), p. 2.

2. L. Stufflebeam, W. J. Foley, W. J. Gephast, E. G. Guba, R. L. Hammond, H. O. Merriman, M. M. Provus, *Educational Evaluation and Decision-Making* (Bloomington, Ind.: Phi Delta Kappan National Study Committee on Education, 1971), p. 17.

3. M. Scriven, "Pros and Cons about Goal-Free Evaluation," *Evaluation Comment* 3, no. 4 (1972): 1-4.

4. Blaine R. Worthen and James R. Sanders, *Educational Evaluation: Theory and Practice* (Belmont, Calif.: Wadsworth Publishing Co., Inc., 1973), pp. 209-217.

## SUGGESTED READINGS

Chase, Clinton I. *Elementary Statistical Procedures.* New York: McGraw-Hill Book Co., 1967.

Gorden, Raymond L. *Interviewing: Strategy, Techniques, and Tactics.* Homewood, Ill.: The Dorsey Press, 1975.

Knox, Alan B., ed. *Assessing the Impact of Continuing Education.* San Francisco: Jossey-Bass, Inc., Number 3, 1979.

Koosis, Donald J. *Statistics.* New York: John Wiley & Sons, Inc., 1972.

Le Breton, Preston; Bryant, Vernon; Zweizig, Douglas; Middaugh, Dana; Bryant, Anita Gras; and Corbett, Tricia (eds.) *The Evaluation of Continuing Education for Professionals: A Systems View.* Seattle: The University of Washington, 1979.

# Chapter 10

# Accreditation/Approval of Continuing Education and Staff Development Activities

Accreditation of continuing education and staff development activities is a process whereby the approval body grants public recognition that such programs have met its established standards for excellence. The accreditation of continuing education in nursing is accomplished primarily through the mechanism established by the American Nurses' Association (ANA).[1] The authority to establish such a mechanism resulted from a resolution adopted at the 1974 ANA House of Delegates, which directed the ANA board of directors to "establish a system of accreditation of continuing education programs in nursing." The Commission on Nursing Education is the structural unit in the ANA responsible for the establishment and maintenance of the accreditation mechanism.

The accreditation model includes a National Accreditation Board that has overall responsibility for the development, implementation, and evaluation of the process. The three regional accrediting committees (RACs)—Eastern, Central, and Western—are responsible to the board and oversee the application of a uniform process of approval. The RACs accredit State Nurses' Associations (SNAs) as providers or approvers of continuing education. As an approved provider, an SNA has obtained recognition that it has the ability to meet criteria established by the ANA in conducting a total program of planning, implementing, and evaluating continuing education in nursing. Accreditation as an approver means that the SNA can approve the programs of other sponsors or of its constituents (district nurses' associations). Access to the ANA accreditation model thus is guaranteed for program sponsors at the local level.

Others eligible for accreditation as providers of continuing education include colleges and universities, national nursing and specialty nursing organizations, federal nursing services, and state boards of nursing. Others eligible for accreditation as approval bodies include state boards of nursing, national specialty nursing organizations, or federal nursing services that may approve the individual courses of their constituent associations.

In addition, the regional committees accredit programs leading to certificates as nurse practitioners in various areas of practice such as pediatrics, gerontology, or obstetrics/gynecology. Standards and criteria have been established that these programs must meet to obtain accreditation.

Other sponsors of programs that may receive approval from a regional accrediting committee include commercial products companies such as pharmaceutical firms that have as their major focus something other than continuing education. These companies may apply for approval of an educational offering on an individual basis or of their continuing education program, defined as a planned, organized effort directed toward accomplishing major objectives. A program can include many segments that are described as educational offerings or courses.

## ACCREDITING BODIES' ROLE DEFINED

The organization, purpose, and functions of the National Accreditation Board and the regional accrediting committees are defined specifically as to the design, implementation, and evaluation of the approval process. Membership on both national and regional bodies generally includes:

- representatives of continuing education or staff development in nursing
- representatives from nursing practice, who must spend a specified amount of time providing direct service to patients in order to be eligible to serve
- an individual with expertise in credentialing, such as certification or licensure
- a consumer of nursing services, usually an individual not employed in the health care system
- an individual designated as a member at large, or one not represented in the other categories, who may be selected to provide another area of expertise (nursing service administration or a faculty member in a program of basic educational preparation for nursing).

Each accredited SNA has established an approval mechanism that follows standards and criteria established in the accreditation model. The criteria an SNA must meet to be accredited as an approval body involve its philosophy, organizational structure, resources (both in personnel and financial), records and reports, approval process, and evaluation. While all of the criteria are specified in some detail, several are identified as essential components:

- identification of an SNA structural unit responsible for the approval process, with clearly defined selection criteria for its members

- selection criteria for members of the body to whom sponsors may appeal adverse decisions

- clearly apparent financial resources, with evidence that the organization responsible for implementation of the approval process also is fiscally responsible for it

- confidentiality of records and reports, which must be stored in such a manner as to permit their easy retrieval

- an evaluation tool based on criteria for the approval process.

Accreditation means that an SNA must have standards and criteria for approval of continuing education activities that comply with those established by the ANA. The ANA standards address:

- assessment of the learning needs of the potential participants
- the design of the educational activity
- implementation of the program design
- the program's objectives
- teaching methodologies
- evaluation of both the process and outcome of the offering
- the recordkeeping system
- organizational resources, human and financial

## APPROVAL OF ACTIVITY

Criteria for SNA approval of an educational offering are based upon the ANA standards. The criteria usually specify such aspects of the standards as:

## Objectives

1. Relevance to current nursing practice

- Under the stated objectives, will the learners:

—acquire new knowledge and skills?
—update knowledge and skills?
—prepare for reentry into practice?
—make a transition from one area of practice to another?
—acquire greater depth of knowledge and skills in one particular area of nursing?
—implement meaningful change both in their own practice and throughout the health care delivery system?
—assume responsibility for personal and professional development?
—improve the ability of other health care workers to meet the specific needs of the public served by the health agency?
—promote and support innovation and creativity in health services?

- Is clinical experience planned to help the participants effect changes in their nursing practice based upon the application of increased knowledge and/or skills?

2. Needs assessment

- Is there substantiation of the need for the educational activity?

3. Measurement (behavior)

- Does the program outline include behaviorally stated objectives?

4. Attainment in time allotted (clinical and/or theory)

- Does the format indicate sufficient time for achieving the desired clinical competencies?

## Content

1. Relation to objectives

- Are content and learning experiences planned to meet these objectives?

- Does the outline reflect consideration of the stated level of participants in its objectives and content?

- Is clinical experience directed toward attainment of specific results, with participants given the opportunity to determine their own objectives for learning in the clinical setting?

2. Planning in logical order

## Method

1. Relation to objectives

   - Does the activity outline reflect the format and teaching methodology?

   - Are the educational methods and materials selected for effectiveness in achieving the objectives and do they reflect variety?

   - Is clinical experience planned to help the participants integrate the knowledge and skills acquired in class?

2. Participation

   - Does the outline reflect methods of active participation?

   - Is clinical experience (actual or simulated) used as a learning method for clinically oriented courses?

   - Have clinical facilities that will be used been identified?

3. Appropriateness for level

   - Does the outline reflect consideration of the stated level of participant in the methods of teaching?

## Evaluation

1. Relation to objectives

   - Are the program objectives considered when participants evaluate the course?

   - Are the evaluation tools appropriate for the program?

   - Are evaluation methods designed specifically for the clinical experience and are they related to its objectives?

2. Planned part of offering

   - What is the evaluation plan? Does the plan include a follow-up evaluation when appropriate?

3. Use of evaluation

   - What is the plan for utilizing the evaluation results?

## Faculty and Speakers

1. Academic preparation

   - Are the instructors' backgrounds relevant to the topic or clinical supervision?

   - Are vitae examined for educational credentials (formal and continuing)?

   - Are experts in the specified disciplines involved in the course?

2. Work experience

   - Again, are faculty members' backgrounds relevant to the topic or clinical supervision?

   - Are vitae examined for work experience, expertise, and recognition in the field?

## Planners

1. Representation of intended audience

   - Is a learner designated as a member of the planning committee?

   - Does the committee show evidence of input from disciplines involved in the course?

2. Knowledge of nursing, health care practices, and adult education principles

   - Does the planning committee have members knowledgeable in adult education and appropriate areas of nursing expertise?

   - Are the designated sponsors directly concerned with at least one aspect of programming?

## Facilitation

1. Appropriateness of facilities

   - Achievement of objectives

     —Has the sponsor provided for resources needed to meet the objectives?
     —Are participants in clinical experience functioning as learners rather than as part of the staff?

- Selection of teaching method

    —Is there sufficient space and audiovisual equipment at the facility for the methods to be utilized?

2. Announcement of educational activity

- Level of learner

    —Does the program announcement indicate the level of participants?
    —Does the format specify the number and disciplines to be involved?

- Statement of objectives

    —Do the participants have prior access to the objectives stated in the announcement?

A rating of the extent to which an educational activity may meet these criteria takes various forms.

## WEIGHTED RATING FORM SYSTEM

One way, which has proved to be both valid and reliable through five years of use in Indiana, is a weighted rating form. The form was designed by the Michigan Nurses' Association and adapted for use by the Indiana Statewide Plan for Continuing Education in Nursing in 1975.

### Division into Seven Categories

Seven categories to be considered for review are ranked in order of importance in the weighted rating form. The objectives category receives the highest priority since all else depends upon identification of expected outcomes. Next comes the content, followed by teaching methods. This could be ranked equally with evaluation, but the method involves achieving the objectives and thus is ranked one category higher than evaluation. The faculty is ranked next, followed by the planners, and finally by facilities to be used.

Key factors, ranked in order of importance, are added in each category.

In the first category, objectives, relevancy to current nursing practice is considered most important and is assigned a weight of 4. Need assessment is weighted with a 3, as is measurability. Attainability in the time allotted is the final factor and is weighted with a 2.

In the category of content, relating to objectives is weighted 4, and planning in logical order is 1. In the method category, relating to objectives is weighted 4, active participation 3, and appropriateness to the level of the learner 1.

The evaluation category also includes three key factors: relation to objectives is once again weighted 4, planning 2, and use of evaluation 1.

Faculty members are rated on two key factors, academic preparation and work experience related to the topic, which are equally weighted with 3s.

The planning category is rated next. An equal weighting of 2 is given for the extent to which the planners represent the intended audience and their knowledge of nursing or health care, and principles of adult education.

Finally, the category of facilitation contains four key factors, equally weighted with 1s. These are the extent to which (1) the facilities are appropriate to achieve the objectives, (2) the facilities are appropriate for the teaching method selected, (3) the course announcement includes the level of learner, and (4) the announcement includes a statement of objectives.

On a scale of one to five then, where 5 is excellent, 4 is very good, 3 is acceptable, 2 is fair, and 1 is unacceptable, each key factor is rated. The ranking on the scale of 1-5 is multiplied by the weight of the key factor. The sum of the weighted ratings of each factor is then divided by the best score possible.

In category one, objectives, the best possible factor score is 60, so that is used as the divider. To give the category its appropriate value in relation to all other categories, the factor score is multiplied by the category position. Since category one, objectives, is assigned the highest priority of the seven, the factor score is multiplied by 7. The best possible factor score for the content category is 25, for method 40, for evaluation 35, for faculty and speakers 30, for planners 20, and for facilitation 20. Each of the sums of the key factors is divided by the best possible factor score and then multiplied by the category score, which is 7 for objectives, 6 for content, 5 for method, 4 for evaluation, 3 for faculty and speakers, 2 for planners and 1 for facilitation.

A final percentile score is calculated by adding all seven category scores and dividing by 28. (Twenty-eight is the sum of the rankings of the categories: 7 plus 6 plus 5 plus 4 plus 3 plus 2 plus 1.)

The passing score is the minimum rank of each factor, in this instance a 3, which is acceptable. The passing score turns out to be 60 percent out of a possible 100 percent.

While mathematical rating is not infallible, it would be difficult to arrive at a passing score unless the key categories, such as objectives, content, and method, are rated as acceptable. The use of such a weighted rating method affords some objectivity in the review process.

## Review and Approval Bodies

Most SNAs have identified a group of individuals who are responsible for the review and approval process. These groups have various titles, such as review board, review panel, or committee on approval. They generally are composed of representatives similar to those at the national and regional levels. The sponsor of a course being reviewed for approval is apprised of what information is needed in the application. Generally, the sponsor receives notification that the application has been received for review, and upon completion of the process, is notified whether it has been approved or not. In either case, suggestions for improvement usually are included. In the event the course was not approved, the sponsor is notified of how to appeal.

The review process varies by state, depending on what is involved. Policies and procedures outlining the process are available in advance of the application to the SNA so the sponsor will know what is expected. Often continuing education staff members in an SNA are available to help the sponsor in the planning process and in completing the application for review. Sometimes members of the review group also are available for this purpose. Sponsors find it useful to avail themselves of this help, especially the first time they submit an application. Some SNAs provide model applications to serve as guides.

Review group meetings may be open so that sponsors can attend to learn how their program is analyzed; they should be encouraged to take advantage of this opportunity so they can learn how the criteria are applied.

The time frame for submitting an application also varies by state. Some states require as little as two weeks' lead time before the course is to start, others as much as two months. Most states will not review programs for retroactive approval, so that sponsors' awareness of deadline dates is essential.

Fees for approving courses also vary by state. The average generally is $15 to $20 per activity. Approval usually is for one year, during which the course may be repeated as often as desired. Changes such as in speakers or in content must be reported to the SNA to ensure continued approval.

Some SNAs require some follow-up activity by the sponsor such as sending in a report of attendance, a summary of the participants' evaluations, or other relevant information.

Sponsors eligible for approval through the SNA include hospitals, long-term care agencies, other health care agencies, colleges and universities that do not have ANA accreditation as a provider, and professional education groups whose only product is continuing education.

## PROGRAM APPROVAL

In addition to approving individual courses, many SNAs have established a mechanism to implement total institutional approval. Most such systems are patterned after that developed by the ANA. Criteria for approval of such a continuing education program include the elements shown in Exhibit 10-1.

# Exhibit 10-1 Example of Checklist for Site Visit

**ISPCEN/ISNA**
**Continuing Education Program Approval**
**Site Visitor Check List**

ISNA/SPCEN #

Name of Organization _____

Address/City _____

Site Visitor _____

Date of Site Visit _____

| CRITERIA | REVIEW OF APPLICATION | | | SITE VISIT | |
|---|---|---|---|---|---|
| | Criteria met | Criteria not met | Uncertain | Comments | Decision |
| **A. Philosophy** | | | | | |
| 1. Recent statement of beliefs about nature of continuing education in nursing | | | | | |
| **B. Goals (Purpose)** | | | | | |
| 1. Goals | | | | | |
|   a. Indicate concern for promotion and advancement of health care | | | | | |
|   b. Identify current trends nursing and health care practices | | | | | |
|   c. Indicate evidence of community involvement | | | | | |
|   d. Show evidence of recent updating/revision | | | | | |
|   e. Have evaluation program for attainment | | | | | |
| **C. Organization** | | | | | |
| 1. Structure | | | | | |
|   a. Current table of organization | | | | | |
|   b. Table of organization distinguishes line/reporting relationships | | | | | |
|   c. Organizational structure indicates it is appropriate for implementation of goals/objectives | | | | | |
|   d. Appropriate personnel for administrative positions | | | | | |
|   e. Continuing education unit capable of full continuous uninterrupted operation | | | | | |
|     (1) All persons in the report are part of the unit as in the report | | | | | |
|     (2) Qualifications of participants are current | | | | | |
|     (3) Staff is adequate in qualification and number | | | | | |
| **D. Planning** | | | | | |
| 1. Participants | | | | | |
|   a. Level of learner population identified and described | | | | | |
|   b. Evidence of learner input in the offering planning | | | | | |
|   c. Provisions made to ascertain characteristics of population attending offering | | | | | |
| 2. Method of assessing learner needs is identified | | | | | |
|   a. Learners may attend different sessions of offerings depending on need | | | | | |
|   b. Requests for offerings given consideration | | | | | |
| 3. Scheduling gives consideration to time and location of sessions that serve the learner population | | | | | |

| CRITERIA | REVIEW OF APPLICATION | | | SITE VISIT | |
|---|---|---|---|---|---|
| | Criteria met | Criteria not met | Uncertain | Comments | Decision |
| 4. Evidence of different time slots, distributions and locations convenient to the learner | | | | | |
| 5. Faculty qualified in the subject area and knowledgeable about principles of adult education | | | | | |
| 6. Conflicts of interest avoided | | | | | |
| 7. Co-sponsorship reflects ISNA policy statement | | | | | |
| **E. Content** | | | | | |
| 1. Objectives | | | | | |
|   a. Describe expected learner outcomes and can be evaluated | | | | | |
|   b. Indicate relationship to nursing | | | | | |
|   c. Reflect needs of learners, employers and consumers | | | | | |
| 2. Continuing education offerings | | | | | |
|   a. Designed to improve nursing practice | | | | | |
|   b. Reflect current research | | | | | |
|   c. Have content which relates to the stated philosophy, goals and behavioral objectives | | | | | |
|   d. Relate to former and current offerings | | | | | |
|   e. Demonstrate that learning experiences are appropriate to achieve objectives and<br>(1) are adequate in kind and number<br>(2) can be achieved in the allotted time<br>(3) achievement of objectives can be evaluated post offering<br>(4) show evidence of consultation<br>(5) provision for continuity of staff | | | | | |
| **F. Teaching Methodologies** | | | | | |
| 1. Principles of adult education used in the proposed teaching strategies | | | | | |
|   a. Basic principals assessed from review of past offerings | | | | | |
|   b. Methods appropriate for level of learning | | | | | |
|   c. Approaches related to offering objectives | | | | | |
|   d. Variety of approaches used which involve active learner participation | | | | | |
|   e. Adequate time allotted | | | | | |
| 2. Clinical experiences | | | | | |
|   a. Integrate the knowledge and/or skills gained | | | | | |
|   b. Planned to effect changes in nursing practice based upon application of increased knowledge and/or skills | | | | | |
|   c. Directed toward attainment of specific objectives with participants given opportunity to determine own objectives for learning in clinical setting | | | | | |
|   d. Under supervision of qualified persons | | | | | |
|   e. Participants function as learners rather than as part of staffing pattern of unit | | | | | |
|   f. Evaluation methods designed specifically for clinical experiences and related to clinical experience objectives | | | | | |

**Exhibit 10-1 continued**

| CRITERIA | REVIEW OF APPLICATION | | | SITE VISIT | |
|---|---|---|---|---|---|
| | Criteria met | Criteria not met | Uncertain | Comments | Decision |
| **G. Resources** | | | | | |
| 1. Personnel | | | | | |
| a. Professional staff adequate in number and preparation to carry out organization's objectives related to continuing education in nursing | | | | | |
| (1) Person administratively responsible for continuing education program should be nurse prepared at graduate level, having skills/knowledge regarding adult education | | | | | |
| (2) Instructors with expertise/competence in offering content utilized | | | | | |
| (3) Evidence that program director and faculty collaborate with other nursing faculty, other health discipline faculty, and nonhealth-related groups in planning and developing offerings | | | | | |
| b. Adequate and qualified support staff, including both technical and clinical personnel, available to implement continuing education activities | | | | | |
| c. An advisory committee used: functions stated. If advisory committee not used, mechanism exists for input from consumers | | | | | |
| 2. Financial | | | | | |
| a. Evidence in the budget to provide funds from fees, dues and other sources to conduct continuing education activities | | | | | |
| b. Allocation of funds appears adequate | | | | | |
| 3. Physical Facilities | | | | | |
| a. Adequate physical facilities, including space and equipment, exist | | | | | |
| **H. Appraisal Procedures** | | | | | |
| 1. Procedures are established for evaluation of | | | | | |
| a. Learning outcomes as part of offering | | | | | |
| b. Services, facilities and resources | | | | | |
| c. Effectiveness in relation to improved nursing practice | | | | | |
| 2. Evaluation tools used are objective and valid | | | | | |
| 3. Appraisal procedures for total program are cost effective | | | | | |
| 4. Evaluation data obtained | | | | | |
| **I. Records and Reports** | | | | | |
| 1. Defined standard of measurement in use | | | | | |
| 2. System of record keeping which | | | | | |
| a. Is available or readily retrievable | | | | | |
| b. Avoids duplication | | | | | |
| c. Maintains participants' confidentiality | | | | | |
| d. Contains information about each offering | | | | | |
| (1) Planning Committee | | | | | |
| (2) Minutes of planning meetings | | | | | |
| (3) Offering Flyer | | | | | |
| (4) Offering outline and teaching techniques | | | | | |
| (5) Curriculum vita of faculty | | | | | |
| (6) Summary of offering evaluation | | | | | |

| CRITERIA | REVIEW OF APPLICATION | | | SITE VISIT | |
|---|---|---|---|---|---|
| | Criteria met | Criteria not met | Uncertain | Comments | Decision |
| 3. Retrievable record system regarding participants includes | | | | | |
|   a. Name and address. | | | | | |
|   b. Identification number | | | | | |
|   c. Employment data | | | | | |
|   d. Offering title, date and location | | | | | |
|   e. Contact hours and number of CEU or other measurable unit | | | | | |
|   f. Policy regarding CEU for partial attendance | | | | | |
|   g. Sponsoring agency | | | | | |
|   h. Director for offering | | | | | |
|   i. General content level | | | | | |
|   j. Approval verification | | | | | |
| 4. Offering announcements indicate | | | | | |
|   a. Statement of objectives | | | | | |
|   b. Level of participant | | | | | |
|   c. Kind of participant | | | | | |
|   d. Date, time and place | | | | | |
|   e. Fee structure | | | | | |
|   f. Contact hours or CEU | | | | | |
|   g. Sponsoring agencies | | | | | |
|   h. Faculty | | | | | |

FINAL SUMMARY

Strengths:

Weaknesses:

Recommendations for program improvement/modification:

7/77

*Source:* Reprinted by permission of Indiana Statewide Plan for Continuing Education in Nursing, Indianapolis, ©1977.

## Philosophy

1. The organization has a recent statement of beliefs about the nature of continuing education in nursing.

## Goals (Purpose)

1. There is a statement of the organization's goals. These goals:

- Indicate concern for the promotion and advancement of health care
- Identify current trends in nursing and health care practices
- Indicate evidence of community involvement
- Show evidence of recent updating or revision
- Reflect *or* demonstrate *or* describe an evaluation program for goal attainment

## Organization

1. Structure

- There is a current table of organization
- This table clearly distinguishes line and reporting relationships among professionals, volunteers, and staff
- The description of the structure indicates it is appropriate for implementation of program goals and objectives
- There are appropriate personnel for administrative positions
- The unit that assumes responsibility for continuing education is capable of uninterrupted operation
- All persons in the report are part of that unit
- Qualifications of participants are current as in the report
- Staff is adequate in qualification and number

## Planning

1. Participants

- The level of the target learner population is identified and described

- There is evidence of learner input in the planning stage
- Provisions are made to ascertain characteristics of the population actually attending

2. Method of assessing learner needs is identified

   - Learners may attend different sessions of courses, depending on individual need
   - Requests for programs are given consideration

3. The scheduling of educational activities gives consideration to time and location of sessions that best serve the student population

4. Scheduling of courses provides evidence of different time slots, distributions, and locations convenient to learners

5. Faculty members are qualified in their subjects and knowledgeable about principles of adult education

6. Conflicts of interest have been avoided

7. Cosponsorship agreements for courses reflect the ANA policy statement

## Content

1. Objectives

   - The objectives describe the expected outcomes for learners and can be evaluated
   - The objectives indicate the relationship to nursing and the bodies of knowledge that contribute to current or emerging patterns of nursing practice

2. Continuing education activities

   - These are designed to improve nursing practice
   - They reflect results of current research findings
   - Their content clearly relates to the stated philosophy, goals, and behavioral objectives

- They show evidence of relationship to former and current courses
- They demonstrate that learning experiences are appropriate to achieve the objectives and:

    —are adequate in kind and number
    —can be achieved in the allotted time
    —can evaluate the achievement of objectives after the course
    —show evidence of consultation as needed if available
    —provide for continuity of staff

## Teaching Methodologies

1. Principles of adult education are used in the proposed teaching strategies

    - Basic principles can be assessed from a review of past programs
    - Methods are appropriate for the level of learning
    - Approaches are related to objectives
    - A variety of approaches have been used that involve active learner participation
    - Adequate time has been allotted

2. When clinical experiences are an integral part of a course or workshop, they meet the following criteria:

    - They are planned to help the participants integrate the knowledge and skills they have acquired
    - They are planned to help the participants effect changes in their nursing practice based upon the application of their increased knowledge and skills
    - They are directed toward attainment of specific objectives, giving nurses the opportunity to determine their own objectives for learning in the clinical setting
    - They are under the supervision of qualified persons
    - They provide for participants in clinical experiences to function as learners rather than as part of the staffing pattern of the unit
    - Their evaluation methods include tools designed specifically for the clinical experiences that are related to the objectives

## Resources

1. Personnel

   - The organization uses professional staff members who are adequate in number and in preparation to carry out objectives specifically related to continuing education in nursing

     —The person administratively responsible for the program should be a nurse prepared at the graduate level and having skills and knowledge about adult education.
     —Instructors with expertise and competence in presenting subject matter are utilized
     —There is evidence that the program director and faculty collaborate with other nursing faculty members, other health discipline faculty persons, and nonhealth-related groups in planning and developing programs

   - Adequate and qualified support staff, including both technical and clinical personnel, are available to implement educational activities

   - An advisory committee is used and its functions are stated clearly; if such a committee is not used, a mechanism such as telephone call-ins or surveys exists for input from consumers of the services

2. Financial

   - The budget provides funds from fees, dues, and other sources to support the program

   - Allocation of funds appears adequate

3. Physical facilities

   - Adequate physical facilities, including space and equipment, exist and are used by the organization in program activities

## Appraisal Procedures

1. Procedures are established:

   - For evaluation of learning outcomes as a planned part of each activity

   - For evaluation of services, facilities, and resources

   - For evaluation of course effectiveness in relation to improved nursing practice

## Records and Reports

1. There is a defined standard of measurement in use

2. There is a system of recordkeeping that:

   - Is available or readily retrievable

   - Avoids duplication

   - Maintains participants' confidentiality

   - Contains information about each course

     —Planning committee
     —Minutes of planning meetings
     —Course flier
     —Course outline and teaching techniques
     —Curriculum vitae of faculty
     —Summary of evaluation

3. There is a retrievable record system regarding participants, including:

   - Name and address of participant

   - Identification number

   - Employment data

   - Course title, date(s), and location

   - Contact hours and number of Continuing Education Units (CEU) or other measurable units

   - Policy regarding CEU for partial attendance

   - Sponsoring agency

   - Program director

   - General content level

   - Approval verification

4. There are course announcements that indicate:

   - Statement of objectives

   - Level of participant

- Kind of participant
- Date, time, and place
- Fee structure
- Contact hours or CEU
- Sponsoring agencies
- Faculty

Policies and procedures for program approval vary by state, as do those for individual class approvals. An application for program approval is submitted, attesting to the sponsor's ability to plan, implement, and evaluate continuing education activities. A track record of successful workshops, courses, or symposiums may be a prerequisite for submitting an application.

## The Site Visit

Generally, approval also involves a site visit by members of the review group to validate, clarify, and amplify the information in the application. Site visitors usually are from an organization similar to the one to be visited. For example, someone from a hospital rather than a university would be chosen to visit a hospital. Most visitors are selected for their expertise in continuing education, although representatives from nursing practice may be chosen, particularly when a service agency such as a hospital is being visited. The visitors usually are given a checklist so the visit will be organized (Exhibit 10-1) to facilitate the collection of information based on the criteria. The site reviewers analyze the application several times before going to the institution and identify areas on which they need more information.

The reviewers meet the night before the site visit to compare notes and plan the visit. A tentative agenda has been prepared, usually by the individual designated by the approval body as the team leader. This agenda has been shared with the institution in advance, but is considered tentative by both groups, since the night-before review may necessitate some changes.

The site visitors' tentative agenda usually consists of a series of meetings with (1) the continuing education program director, (2) persons having administrative responsibility for that program, such as a hospital director of the department of education or director of nursing, (3) members of planning committees for educational activities, (4) faculty members, (5) nurse participants, and (6) departmental support staff. The visitors often will request a tour of the institution, particularly so they can see its educational resources. They review reports and the recordkeeping system. At several points during the day, the visitors may request to be alone to review materials, discuss the site visit process, and determine additional information needed.

At the conclusion of the visit, the team prepares an oral report for the applicant summarizing its findings. The report does not give an indication whether the accrediting body will approve the program or not. Clarification of concerns should be attended to before the group leaves. There should be provision for the sponsor to evaluate the site visitors as well.

There is a certain amount of anxiety on both sides. This is natural and, while it should be acknowledged, it should not be dwelled upon. Nor should anxiety be allowed to interfere with the site visit process in any way. Social amenities can help reduce anxiety but should not take precedence over the business at hand. The process can be exhausting for everyone; however, it should prove to be an educational process.

The site visitors prepare a report for the approval body, which makes the ultimate decision based upon site visitors' findings and recommendation. The decision is communicated to the sponsor. In the event a program is not approved, assistance should be available so that the sponsor can work toward meeting the criteria. The sponsor also should be apprised about the appeal process for applications that are not approved.

## Fees for Approval

Fees for the program approval process vary from state to state; the average is $100 to $200, plus the expenses of the site visitors. Attempts usually are made to obtain visitors from near the sponsoring agency to minimize expenses.

The period of approval may vary from one to four years, with the average two years.

## Follow-Up Activities

There are varying follow-up requirements for approved programs. Sponsors may be asked to send in a calendar of their proposed continuing education courses for a specified period. Approval may require the submission of quarterly or annual progress reports and records of attendance or summaries of evaluations.

Reapplication following an initial period of approval may require that the entire process be repeated, including the site visit. The approved program may be requested to submit samples of successful activities, plus a narrative describing any changes based on the site visitors' recommendations, with the reapproval decision made on the basis of that information.

Most SNAs have established a system for monitoring programs when complaints are received. Guidelines for monitoring should be shared with sponsors who might become involved. Expenses for monitoring visits usually are the financial responsibility of the institution being surveyed. In most instances, a close working relationship between approval body and approved program will prevent the necessity for monitoring.

## Reciprocity of Approvals

Approval of a program by an SNA that is accredited as an approval body by the ANA means that there is reciprocity of that decision among 21 similarly accredited SNAs. In the event that an activity is sponsored by an accredited SNA, or a college or university that has been accredited as a provider, again there is reciprocity among all bodies that are part of the ANA approval mechanism.

One of the stipulations when accreditation or approval is granted to an applicant agency is that all promotional materials carry an announcement to that effect. Thus, it is easy for nurses to identify which continuing education activities have the guarantee of quality from their professional association that consequently will be reciprocal among many states.

## THE CONTINUING EDUCATION UNIT

Participation in courses often is measured by the Continuing Education Unit (CEU), which is defined as "ten contact hours of participation in an organized continuing education experience under responsible sponsorship, capable direction, and qualified instruction." The CEU was developed by a national task force after the need for a standard for measurement of nonacademic education was identified.[2] The task force later stated that CEU is the preferred term in both singular and plural use.

The CEU measures participation in nonacademic credit activities in much the same way as the semester, trimester, or quarter-hour marks participation in academic credit activities. The CEU awarded by general continuing education departments in colleges or universities often are equated with the FTE (full-time equivalent) for funding purposes. A contact hour is defined as a typical 50-minute classroom period. If the educational offering is not held in the typical classroom setting, the sponsor may choose to calculate a contact hour as a 60-minute clock hour. Clinical experience contact hours usually are calculated on a 2:1 ratio, that is, two clock hours or 120 minutes of clinical experience is equivalent to one contact hour.

It is the responsibility of the sponsor to award the appropriate number of contact hours or CEU. The accrediting body has the responsibility to approve the awarding of contact hours or CEU that indicate that the quality standards have been met.

## Requirements for Awarding CEU

Any sponsor can award CEU. The only requirement is that the sponsor adhere to the guidelines established by the national task force. In 1977 the Council on the Continuing Education Unit was formed to carry on the work of the national task force, which then was dissolved. The council has maintained the same standards for awarding CEU; it also has designed a certification mark that sponsors may use if they are institutional members of the council. All sponsors, however, may use the CEU as a unit of measurement provided they:

- have an identifiable educational arm that is administered by professional staff

- maintain administrative control of all of the continuing education activities they sponsor

- provide or arrange for appropriate educational facilities, including the locations in which programs are held, and related resources (materials or equipment)

- maintain individual records of participation on a permanent basis that participants can request if needed

The Council on the Continuing Education Unit established program criteria that must be met—among them that:

- the activity is conducted under responsible sponsorship, capable direction, and qualified instruction

- the activity is planned on the basis of the needs of the target audience

- a clear statement of purpose and goals is prepared for each educational activity

- qualified instructors conduct the course

- there are specific performance requirements for participants to establish eligibility to earn CEU

- registration forms contain enough information to permit permanent records to be kept

- records must be kept to verify completion by each participant who is awarded CEU

- the course or workshop is evaluated in terms of its design and operation.

There are some events for which CEU should not be awarded: courses for academic credit, committee meetings, entertainment or recreational activities such as travel groups, or high school equivalency programs. Another activity that does not qualify for CEU is being faculty members in an educational activity, even though they may spend considerable time preparing the material they are to present. CEU are not awarded for the preparation, presentation, or publication of papers and reports, nor for work or on-the-job experience. Other units must be designed to measure these activities, if appropriate and necessary. Only individuals who participate in the courses are eligible to receive CEU.

When calculating the CEU to be awarded, only the time spent in the educational experience should be considered. Time spent in making announcements, introductions, lunches, coffee breaks, and visiting exhibits, for example, are not included.

Only complete instructional hours are counted. When calculating CEU hours, rounding up is inappropriate. If, for example, a course runs 5½ hours, then .5 CEU are awarded; the time is not rounded up to .6 CEU. Nor, if the program runs 5½ hours, are .55 CEU awarded since only complete instructional hours are calculated.

## Proof of Completion

The council recommends that CEU be awarded only upon proof of satisfactory completion of the course. That proof may be the passing of a posttest, an evaluation of the program, or whatever demonstration of completion is deemed appropriate by the director. Only individuals who complete the requirements satisfactorily should be awarded CEU. If the award is based only on attendance, then prorating is appropriate, but the course objectives generally are not met if the nurse does not participate in the entire program. If a notice that attendance is necessary at all sessions to receive CEU is included with the course publicity, participants will be forewarned that the unit will be awarded only at the conclusion of the entire program.

The approval of educational activities by an ANA-accredited SNA for which the sponsor awards CEU indicates that the program meets the criteria established by the National Task Force and the Council on the Continuing Education Unit and the standards for quality continuing education as established by the professional organization for nurses. Such indications of quality are essential in assuring consumers of nursing care services that the continuing education in which practitioners participate meets established standards.

## OTHER APPROVAL SYSTEMS

Another group with a well-established approval system for continuing education is the National Federation of Licensed Practical Nurses, Inc. (NFLPN). At the NFLPN convention in 1974, its House of Delegates adopted the CEU standards to measure the participation of licensed practical nurses (L.P.N.s) in continuing education. In addition to the CEU requirements that the activity be an organized experience, under responsible sponsorship, capable direction, and qualified instruction, the NFLPN included criteria on appropriate planning, a purpose, rationale and goals, instructional methods, instructor qualifications, performance requirements, registration and recordkeeping, evaluation and verification of completion.

The NFLPN system for CEU approval is centralized at the national level. Providers of continuing education apply to the association for approval, using application forms supplied by the NFLPN and following its policies and procedures. Upon approval, a process that takes approximately 60 days, a permanent number is assigned to the activity. This number appears on a participant report form that all L.P.N.s in attendance must sign if they wish to have the approved CEU recorded in the NFLPN national data bank. The course provider then verifies completion by L.P.N.s who signed the attendance report form before it is sent back to the national headquarters. The CEU for each individual L.P.N. are entered into the data bank and periodic transcripts of cumulative continuing education activity are made available.

Information about activities that have been approved is stored in the computer so that statistical data on major program areas, providers, and length of programs can be retrieved and reported.

The fee for CEU approval is reasonable. CEU are recorded free for members of the NFLPN and its constituent state associations, but there is a charge for nonmembers. Transcripts of continuing education participation are sent free once a year; additional transcripts can be obtained at a minimal charge when needed by the individual L.P.N.

Many national nursing specialty organizations have systems for continuing education approval. Many of these have been accredited by the American Nurses' Association to provide approved continuing education activities and to approve those of their constituents.[3] Some of the organizations accredited through the ANA mechanism are:

- American Association of Nephrology Nurses and Technicians
- American Association of Occupational Health Nurses
- Association of Operating Room Nurses, Inc.
- Association of Rehabilitation Nurses

- Emergency Department Nurses Association

- Nurses' Association of the American College of Obstetricians and Gynecologists

Professional associations and organizations for health care workers other than nurses also have established standards and criteria for approval of continuing education activities. The appropriate organization should be contacted to obtain information about its approval process.

The involvement of professional associations and organizations for nurses and other health care practitioners in the provision and approval of continuing education is an indication of commitment to the concept of lifelong learning. Participation in continuing education is one means by which nurses and other health care workers can maintain currency and competency in their practice and meet the standards for practice established by their profession.

The profession, then, assumes the responsibility for ensuring that the continuing education in which the practitioner participates meets standards for both educational and professional excellence. To this end, the practice of nurses and others will be enhanced, resulting in the ultimate improvement of health care services for the citizens of the nation.

---

**NOTES**

1. American Nurses' Association, *Accreditation of Continuing Education in Nursing* (Kansas City, Mo.: American Nurses' Association, 1975), p. 2.

2. The Council on the Continuing Education Unit, *Criteria and Guidelines for Use of the Continuing Education Unit* (Silver Spring, Md.: Council on the Continuing Education Unit, 1979), pp. 1-28.

3. American Nurses' Association, *Directory of Accredited Organizations, Approved Programs/ Offerings, and Accredited Continuing Education Certificate Programs Preparing Nurse Practitioners* (Kansas City, Mo.: American Nurses' Association, 1980), pp. 13-14.

---

**SUGGESTED READINGS**

American Nurses' Association. *Continuing Education in Nursing: An Overview.* Kansas City, Mo.: American Nurses' Association, 1976.

American Nurses' Association. *Guidelines for Staff Development.* Kansas City, Mo.: American Nurses' Association, 1976.

# Index

## A

Accessibility to classes, 58
Accreditation. *See also* Approval bodies

body
    philosophy of program and, 26-28
    role of, 234-39
CEU and, 253-55
evaluation and, 218-19, 222
overview of, 233-34
program approval and, 241-53
program of National League for Nursing and, 106
weighted rating form system and, 239-41
Activity approval, 235-39
Administration staffing, 30-33
Adult learners, 5-8
    aspects of learning environment and, 8-13
    basic concepts and, 13-14
    as change agents, 8
    fears of, 7
    as individuals, 14-15
    learning styles and, 7-8
    learning techniques and, 130
    self-concept of nurses and, 6-7

teachers' relationship to, 13-18
Advanced study, objectives and, 122-23
Advertising, 62-63
Advisory committees, 34-36
    group discussion/learning needs and, 85
Affective domain, classifying objectives and, 112, 121
After-the-fact awareness strategy, 4
AIDA formula, brochures, and, 67-69
*American Journal of Nursing,* 130
American Nurses' Association
    accreditation and, 28, 233, 235, 241, 256-57
    lifelong learning and, 1-2
    reciprocity of approval and, 253
    self-directed learning and, 146-47, 149-50
Anticipatory strategies, 3-4
Anxiety
    of adult learners, 7
    evaluation and, 222
    site visits and, 252
    of test experience, 212
Appraisal procedures, approval and, 249

# About the Authors

BELINDA E. PUETZ, R.N., PH.D., formerly was Project Director of the Indiana Statewide Plan for Continuing Education in Nursing (ISPCEN) and now is Director of Continuing Education, Indiana State Nurses' Association, Indianapolis.

FAYE L. PETERS, R.N., M.S.ED., is Coordinator of Continuing Education in Nursing at the Columbus Campus of Indiana University-Purdue University at Indianapolis, and a member of the faculty of the Indiana University School of Nursing in Indianapolis.